T0260178

Cancer in the Lives of Older Americans

Cancer in the Lives of Older Americans

Blessings and Battles

Sarah H. Kagan, Ph.D., R.N.

PENN

University of Pennsylvania Press

Philadelphia

Published by
University of Pennsylvania Press
Philadelphia, Pennsylvania 19104-4112

Printed in the United States of America on acid-free paper

10 9 8 7 6 5 4 3 2 1

Library of Congress Cataloging-in-Publication Data

Kagan, Sarah H. (Sarah Hope)
   Cancer in the lives of older Americans : blessings and battles/Sarah H. Kagan.
      p. cm.
   Includes bibliographical refernces and index.
   ISBN 978-0-8122-4143-3 (alk. paper)
1. Geriatric oncology—United States. 2. Cancer—Psychological aspects—United States. 3. Older people—Diseases—United States. I. Title.
   [DNLM: 1. Neoplasms—psychology—United States. 2. Aged—United States. 3. Social Isolation—psychology—United States. QZ 200 K142c 2009]
RC281.A34.K33 2009
618.97'6994—dc22   2009004267

To Mrs. Eck, who transformed
a few chapters into a book
with her grace and insight

To my niece, Ella Rose,
and my nephews, Reid and Benjamin,
for all that they are

Contents

Introduction: Finding My Way   1

1 Champagne and Hot Dogs   9

2 Being Old, Having Cancer   25

3 Paradox: Cancer and Aging in America   38

4 Scientific Import and Influence   49

5 Language Lessons   65

6 Aesthetics of Being and Having   76

Epilogue: Not a Denial of the Fact of Death, a Denial of Death Now   87

Postscript: Completed   95

Notes   99

References   103

Index   107

Acknowledgments   111

Introduction
Finding My Way

Shortly after New Year's Day of 2006, I found myself on a street in a small town in New Jersey, a quintessentially American street in a typical American town. Even though the town is a short drive from a big city—just off the main commercial thoroughfare—a bedroom suburb lost in an array of similar places across the sprawling American urban landscape, emotionally this street in this town is deeply and personally connected to an enduring image of the American dream. Single-family homes, neat front yards browned by winter, a few children's toys visible in the snowless remains of Christmas celebrations marked this street that was quiet and absent of any traffic at midday. I came to this neighborhood, a neighborhood that seems familiar in the ubiquitous sense of attaining the suburban version of the American dream, to meet a woman who I think embodies what it means to be old and have cancer in America today. I am a nurse who specializes in helping older patients who have cancer understand and manage the experience of cancer. Mrs. Eck is as much everywoman as she is enduringly and impressively herself. Her story, as she tells it, reveals much of what I seek to dissect and analyze from a societal level in a personal odyssey that affirms relationships, values, and perspective. Mrs. Eck's exploration of her family, her faith, and her outlook is centrally illustrative of the themes, concerns, conflicts, and paradox our society faces in understanding the increasingly common experience of what it means to be old and have cancer in America today.

I arrived at the house that Mrs. Eck has shared with her husband of sixty-one years since they purchased it from her parents. She and Mr. Eck moved in a few years after they married, the memory of World War II still fresh in their minds, the promise of family in their future. One of Mrs. Eck's sons, Joe, and his partner, Wayne, were expecting me. Joe, Wayne, and I knew the same editor, a fact that brought me to meet with Mrs. Eck on this mild winter day. Our connection through this editor resulted in a far more common one: Advancing age is the single greatest risk factor for cancer. The older you are, the more likely you are to be diagnosed with cancer. It is a simple enough equation that renders incredibly intricate, nuanced consequences. As our society ages, more and more families share the journey in which the Ecks find themselves immersed. However, unlike the abstract notion of what it must be to be old and have cancer, each of these families—like the Eck family—understands this experience as highly personal and indelibly particular. They are families with generations of history, individual identities, shared understandings, interactions both comforting and provocative, and knowledge of each member of their family that is irreplaceable—for better or worse, but in cases where older family members are ill and need assistance, generally better. Their family story of an older loved one facing cancer was at once illustrative of, and far more profound than, the social discourse and paradox I sought to represent in a series of chapters for this book.

Mrs. Eck's story is where this book begins, and in a way, hers is where this book ends, as her story becomes emblematic of the challenges, triumphs, and everyday lives that many older people who have cancer live each day. The book's genesis reaches back to my first book, *Older Adults Coping with Cancer: Integrating Cancer into a Life Mostly Lived* (Kagan 1997). In the process of researching that book, I found myself in a place that so many young and midlife adults do: I was caring for my Aunt Barbara— my mother's older sister—who had been diagnosed with melanoma in October 1992 just after her sixty-second birthday. Barbara was barely old chronologically and not at all typically old in the way she lived her life. She had lived a normally varied life with ups and downs, and her way of living her daily life revealed that place in life, the cumulative knowing of that life, and the expectations of life events in anticipated retirement and family milestones. Barbara's diagnosis caused my academic and professional interests to collide with my personal life. I took a leave from my work to care for her and learned firsthand the trials, frustrations, and even some satisfactions and gratifications as she received care at a major academic cancer center. She had a primary care provider in the community outside that academic system. Her friends, her brother, my cousins, and I all created an immediate web of instrumental care and emotional support around her. We tried to cushion her and ourselves from byproducts of the unexpected—her disease, its abrupt emergence (she was diagnosed after having a seizure at work one afternoon in October), her prognosis, and her daily life overtaken by decreasing capacity and apparently endless health care encounters.

There was a point where Mrs. Eck told me in our interview of the moment when she overheard some physicians talking about her grave prognosis in very frank terms. They evidently spoke unaware that she could hear them. While I did not even consider the parallel during my time with Mrs. Eck, her story brought me back to a moment in late 1992 when Aunt Barbara called and told me, "My doctor [her primary care physician, not her oncologist] told me I am going to die. What will I do?" While Barbara thought it an appropriate pronouncement—she believed in the sanctity of the role of the physician and had trusted this physician implicitly—she rationalized her emotional devastation by thinking through her intellectual understanding of the disease. I called her primary care physician and explained her devastation, never knowing what he made of our interaction but wanting desperately to convey her experience for his discernment. In addition to some emotional recompense for Barbara, I wanted this physician to understand the consequences of his prognostication so that other families might not feel the enduring sting of such words without context or caveat. The pronouncement of Barbara's death was beyond my point, as I think it was for Mrs. Eck when she overheard the similar prognostication she described to me. In any event, telephoned anticipation of Barbara's death came many months too early. My sole focus in resolving our distress and in educating her physician was Barbara's life, not her death. I wanted desperately as both niece and nurse to sort through how I could help her go on living in a way that she desired and that was free of impositions from well-meaning people like her physician who forgot to ask what she wanted and how she wanted it. This general quest has become a long-standing imperative individualized to patients and their families for whom I care in my practice.

Mrs. Eck brought me full circle, too, in recalling how much I learned from Barbara's experience of comfortable relationships with her oncology team and the gratification that comfort brought me. Remembering the superlative kindness of her oncology fellow (a junior physician in training), the remarkable warmth and attention of her radiation oncologist and the entire radiation team, and the incredible humanity of her visiting nurse still brings me to tears, years after her death. They are tears of appreciation and remembrance of the overwhelming grief they assuaged. Remembrance of relationships that these clinicians had with both my Aunt Barbara and me overrides the still-vivid challenges of co-ordinating her care, unexpectedly harsh interactions, and observation of the sheer hard labor of having cancer when your body has aged sufficiently to lose some of its innate reserve. Ours was a positive family experience of an older loved one living with cancer. Her care was very good, her daily life was what she wanted it to be under the circumstances, and she died as she lived—well, deliberately, and in control. Ours too, like the Ecks', was a very American story of being old and having cancer, although the details, the time, and the place were very different.

The collision that Barbara's diagnosis created in my life—the serious illness of a loved person who had fostered my development in a critical time of my life crashing perilously into the practice of the profession her support enabled me to follow—shattered the ease of that practice and the surety of what I thought I knew. All of this reflection and the sense of disruption that instigated it were, in retrospect, not only understandable but also normal and even healthy. At the time Barbara was diagnosed, I had practiced oncology nursing for just six years. I loved my work and deeply enjoyed varied connections with patients, families, and colleagues—so much so that I pursued graduate studies focused specifically on older adults and especially on older adults who have cancer. Those older people and the way in which I saw them live their lives touched me. I learned from them maxims that I use to coach other patients to this very day. But the maxims were impossible to see without the personal shattering aspects of the professional and consequent reflection to abstract lessons learned.

In a larger existential sense, the collision forced me off the path I thought I saw before me. That path was a peaceful life in practice, in the general direction of my interests in gerontology and oncology but without any driving passion or particular mission. I was left fumbling, searching for another path and a new direction. As with so many devastating life events, I was pushed to a place of reconstructing meaning in my daily life. I began to and still do spend endless time thinking and talking—with those who will engage with me—about myriad facets of the experience of being old—old like Barbara, old in so many other ways of being and meaning—and having cancer. The nature of what it means to be old compels my attention almost constantly. While the state of being old is commonly discussed as an absolute, it is in reality a layered, evanescent flow of human experience. What is old today is glamorized in media analyses of social change tomorrow. A person does not, for example, arise from bed on the morning of a sixtieth or sixty-fifth birthday suddenly old, nor does one become a different person on that particular birthday. Yet social representations of being old clearly connote a moment on which that existence of old age hinges and in which the old become definably different people. My progressive conversation with people who would be judged older by some social standard, whether chronological, functional, or even existential, underscores the nature of aging and of aging in place and situation. I rally against the social notion of distinguishing the old by accounting for difference, choosing instead to see the less visible perpetuation of self and identity with their iterative developmental changes. As a result, my general interests in working with older people who have cancer have evolved. These interests have moved toward a quest to better and more discretely discover how cancers infiltrate my patients' lives both literally—as cancers do—and figuratively, and the ways in which my patients and their lives are altered and are constant.

Many cancers suffered by older adults have caught my attention in the intervening years since Barbara was diagnosed with cancer. Melanoma, the disease Barbara suffered from, and other skin cancers; breast and gynecological cancers such as that of the ovary; and gastrointestinal cancers, such as the diagnosis of pancreatic cancer Mrs. Eck received and the more common diagnosis of colorectal cancer, are diffused throughout the experience of older adults I meet in my daily practice and ongoing inquiry. Breast and colorectal cancers are two of the four most common cancers in our society (Jemal et al. 2005). Cancers of the lung and prostate complete the group—all cancers seen largely in older adults (Jemal et al. 2005). Increasingly, cancers of the head and neck, which are rather rare in the United States but profoundly influence the body, psyche, and soul of those who live with and around them, consume much of my attention (Jemal et al. 2005). They are all cancers—grouped biologically—but they are as individual as the lives they alter. Everything from the symptoms they cause and the treatments they require to the personal introspection and socially mediated perceptions they beget are as unique and simultaneously shared as the older adults, families, friends, and communities living with these illnesses.

Indeed, we do live with cancer in our aging society, from the now ubiquitous bright-yellow *LiveStrong*® wristbands to the very intimate stories of small moments in otherwise normal and quiet lives. This is a new public phenomenon, one that has emerged over the past decade or so. Striving to understand those small moments and the larger alterations in older adults' lives as they are or are not influenced by the experience of being old and having cancer impels me to observe, analyze, and write. In the time since Barbara's death, I have moved from one coast to another, completed research projects transformed by her experience and been informed by a remarkable group of older participants who gave of themselves when I asked, and found life as an academic surprisingly freeing and rewarding as I pursue inquiry and understanding. While I always tell my students that I had said years ago I would never pursue an academic career, I am— years later—happy proof that the adage "never say never" may be expressed in remarkable ways. My academic career is founded upon the broad pursuit of understanding what it means to be old and have cancer, teaching and learning with others in that pursuit, and aiming in my practice to offer some measure of relief and comfort to those who dwell in that state.

My academic life expresses, in large part, the path that I found after the collision of the personal and the professional during Barbara's illness. The path has taken me, in the intervening years, through many events and epiphanies. It has allowed me to meet many people who are living with cancer and other serious illnesses that engender for them complex physical, emotional, spiritual, and social experiences. My patients are young and old. My rather trite joke to explain that I am interested in the span of human life and the process of aging and being old is, "I specialize in the care of older adults. But don't worry, I don't discriminate on the basis of age—I can help you if you are young too!" After that pronouncement, my occasional pediatric patients tend to look at me sideways as their parents ask somewhat puzzled questions. The young adults smile and wonder what I can really do to help them. The people who society would say are "older" offer any number of reactions, from a welcome and welcoming laugh to probing questions about what I think the state of being old really is today. My conversations with patients and their loved ones are imbued with the accreted knowledge of years in practice, the lessons learned from past patients and from my personal life. I often find myself making statements that begin, "People have taught me over the years . . ." and "My patients have helped me learn that . . ." as I counsel and coach. I often remember Barbara as I try to comfort families of patients who are dying when they ask, "What will it [their loved one's death] be like?" and I often begin by saying, "Many people who can anticipate death through an illness like this one die in the way that they lived. Tell me about how your loved one has lived life." It opens a conversation I have found profoundly useful and reflective of understanding that life on this earth, apart from any spiritual beliefs, ends with death. Dying is most certainly not a separate trajectory from that of life.[1]

My path in the past years has also offered unanticipated shifts and new directions in focus and collaborations. A couple of years after I first arrived at the University of Pennsylvania, I stepped backward onto the foot of a reconstructive head-and-neck surgeon while I was instructing one of my students in her care of a patient on my home unit in the Hospital of the University of Pennsylvania. The surgeon, Ara Chalian, did not wince and walk off as he might have done. He laughed at my literal misstep and instead enlisted me to offer an opinion on the care of that patient, whom he was seeing also. The patient was an old man who had been critically ill and had a tracheostomy (a breathing tube inserted through a surgical incision in the neck into the windpipe, or trachea), though not because of cancer. A funny chance meeting and a provocative clinical question began a years-long conversation about living with and treating people who have head and neck cancers and the demands of caring for people whose lives intertwine complex influences of aging, gender, cancer, embodiment,[2] and aesthetics. Ara's colleagueship leveraged an only meager initial interest in head and neck cancers. Care of people with head and neck cancer is now the clinical subspecialty that so powerfully draws much of my interest and attention and has created further collaborations. I am drawn to head and neck cancers not as a group of diseases but because of the way in which these disorders shape people's lives and alter function, identity, and aesthetics.

Any cancer can do as much to alter the life of an afflicted older person. Breast cancers are widely known as diagnoses that reshape women's bodies and lives—some of that reshaping is visible, but much of it is largely invisible as the perception of identity and the self that has been understood for decades is immutably changed. Cancers of the digestive tract—like Mrs. Eck's pancreatic cancer—are less well known than breast cancer. Thus their stamp on the lives of older people is less visible and less available for public discourse such as this book. We can, for example, understand that breast cancer has both public and private ramifications. Media coverage of breast cancer reveals the public implications for women's roles, improvements in breast-conserving surgery, and treatment advances. Social understandings of the breast and some directions in the debate about the manner in which older women's lives and experiences are shifting in an aging society suggest that we can contemplate private and more personal interpretations of breast cancer for older women. Conversely, cancer of the pancreas is less common and more difficult to treat than breast cancer. Mrs. Eck's story of treatment avenues pursued and blocked is not uncommon given the behavior of the disease. Less available media coverage reflects the challenge to successful treatment and the limited options that stem from difficult detection and diagnosis of often advanced cancer—something Mrs. Eck's story reveals to us as well. Finally, the relative degree to which cancers of the digestive tract are discussed in public and championed in media campaigns likely reflects our disinclination to examine the digestive tract, with its mysterious and socially discomfiting emanations. Katie Couric's public voice behind the Entertainment Industry Foundation's initiative called the National Colorectal Cancer Research Alliance is emblematic of how recognition of some of these social forces results in campaigns that target them.[3] Consider, for example, a national news media anchor—Couric—undergoing a colonoscopy to detect colorectal cancer on television. Surmounting several mores about the body, digestion, and defecation in particular is required for the act to achieve its aim of increasing participation in the same test among the audience watching her screening for the most common digestive tract cancer.[4] Arguably, the pancreas has a lower social profile than the colon and rectum in the context of understanding what it is to live with cancer as an older person. Beyond its connections with diabetes mellitus, the pancreas remains a medically suffused void in social conversation. Hence I leapt at the opportunity to interview Mrs. Eck. Her age, life, cancer, and experience represent converging social concerns on which my study centers.

Mrs. Eck's is a singular and personal story in which I hope she shines vividly through as a person with a particular aesthetic and way of being, representing her generation and age as well as the experience of cancer as an older person. How Mrs. Eck reveals meaning in her experience of being old and having cancer is as much her as it is her story of being treated for pancreatic cancer. But it is the lack of social familiarity pancreatic cancer holds that in part allows us to see that experience. More commonly discussed cancers that have the social advantage of being familiar, easily talked about diseases—like breast cancer—may predispose those of us who read and think about being old and having cancer to judge that experience with this advantage in mind. I aim specifically to uncover and highlight less socially known and discussed aspects of being old and having cancer. To achieve this aim, I must in part avoid the familiar, call up the unfamiliar, and contrast the visible and public with the less visible and private. Thus Chapter 6 examines the individual human aesthetic found in embodiment and asks how it is changed by age, gender, and cancer. I strive to reveal this as seen, for example, in the alteration of an older woman's breast in breast cancer treatment or in the fears of an ostomy for colorectal cancer—both generally outdated templates for current treatment of these cancers. The return to consider the aesthetic and social understanding of what it means to be old and have cancer is achieved using the case presented by head and neck cancers, with their uniquely visible effects on the human body and its innate function, as an illustration juxtaposed against the well-known and less visible case of breast cancer. Head and neck cancers are unfamiliar and often affect aesthetics and function in very public ways while breast cancer offers familiarity and a more private impact to illustrate the analysis.

I begin with Mrs. Eck's story, revealing both common and unique themes in her experience, with the aim of setting a human stage for a discussion that often addresses cells and drugs, diagnoses and prognoses without sketching the people who live it. The chapters that follow are a more abstracted discourse on various aspects of what it means to be old and have cancer in our society today. These chapters emerge from my perspective on my practice as a nurse, inquiry, and education and of connections with countless events and individuals who have influenced my thinking. The epilogue returns to Mrs. Eck and her story. Her son, Joe, and his partner, Wayne, and I carried on an extensive conversation around my interview with her. Our dialogue, I think, portrays their hopes and concerns for Mrs. Eck in the context of their relationship with and knowledge of her. Their voices are, as is hers, at once unique and deeply attached to Mrs. Eck and simultaneously illustrative of thoughts and feelings shared by family members of older adults who have cancer across the country. I excerpt and comment upon that conversation to close this discussion of what it means to be old and have cancer in America today.

Chapter 1
Champagne and Hot Dogs

Mrs. Eck is perched on a sofa across from a fire that crackles and smells somehow quintessentially of what this home in this neighborhood on this day should. She is tiny, and my first impression is of her lovely and carefully coiffed red hair and of her tasteful outfit—slacks and a cheerfully cozy sweater—as she greets me rather formally by today's standards of etiquette. We are to have tea and cookies baked by one of her daughters. Mrs. Eck seems precarious and somewhat off balance in the small space she occupies on the sofa. She has a cane—an aluminum adjustable model from a medical equipment supply store, clearly not an affectation but a necessary support—close at hand. I perceive that she is a softly spoken woman, and the sounds of the fire create a washed quiet in the room. I move close to her, sitting carefully on the edge of the sofa cushion, to hear her and gain permission to record her story for this book. In the initial exchange, I tell her that I believe her story might open my book about what it means to be old and have cancer. We talk briefly about how our society seems to struggle with the manner in which her state of being is understood. Her story, I say, will almost certainly ameliorate and teach better than my academic writings would ever do alone. And so convinced, Mrs. Eck begins easily and surprises me with her fluid descriptions and attention to detail.

"Yes, it really started last October, when I—I just was walking down the driveway, and my leg just froze. . . . And I thought, now how am I going to get back to the house? So I pondered that for a bit and then I just started picking it up, picking it up, like this. And I got it so that it [the leg] would move again. That happened to me twice. And then I decided to go to an orthopedist. And they took the X ray, and then the doctor said, you have to have a hip replacement. So I said, well I don't want to have a hip replacement, and, you know, I'm eighty-five years old. And, so they said, well we'll try therapy. So for the whole month of December [2004], I went three days a week through the month, and on my birthday, the thirtieth of December, was my last session. And the therapist said, I don't

usually tell people this, but, she said, you have to have a hip replacement.
So I said I would consider. So we then started searching for a surgeon.
And that got into January [2005]. Suddenly I start itching all over. Every
place. Every place on my body, I could just tear it apart. And I, I've got my
husband going out getting Solarcaine® and spraying me. . . . And nothing is helping. And so at the end of January, my daughter looked at me
one day, I had been to the hairdresser. And she was here, the one that's
the nurse. She looked at me and she said, 'You're yellow.' And she said,
she called the doctor, and he said I was to go to the hospital and have a
blood test taken. So her husband took me the next day to the hospital.
And we're walking in and I said to John, 'This won't be anything, John.
We'll be in and out of here in a minute, they're only going to take some
blood.' Well it wound up I was eight hours in the . . . in the emergency
room, with him still staying there. And I'm saying, 'John, I'm fine, just
leave, you know.' But he wouldn't do it. So it got to be about five o'clock
in the evening, and the doctor finally came and he said, 'We're going to
tuck you in.' So they found a bed for me, and that was my first stay in the
hospital. And then they came in the day after and told me they thought I
had a blocked bile duct, and that I would have to have a stent [small tube
placed in the duct to reopen it] put in. And then I saw them all talking,
and all that, you know. Then I heard one of them say, 'She might die on
the table.' So I, well. . . ."

I interject, shocked that a patient—she might have been my patient—
would have heard such a clinically cold calculation: "You heard that?"

Mrs. Eck replies evenly and without emotion, "I heard that."

"Wow," is all I can inarticulately muster.

Mrs. Eck continues, detailed and precise in how she constructs her
story: "And I thought, oh boy, this is serious, you know. So, but I didn't
say anything anymore about that. And then there was all this discussion
about who was going to put the stent in, and they thought I should go to
Stein Hospital.[1] So they transferred me there, like on a Tuesday night.
And when I got there, they . . . they had me in a room that was a trans-
plant room. All glass and kind of off by its side, self, you know. And I got
settled in there, and I had so many people coming in. I didn't know who
was who. This group, that group, the other group, you know . . . And
then I finally met the doctor who was going to put the stent in the next
day. He was very nice. And he kept telling me, 'Go for the gold, go for
the gold,' you know."

Mrs. Eck laughs, and I ask, "What did he mean by that?"

Mrs. Eck does not really reply to my question and instead picks up the
trail of her story. "And I didn't even know, really, what was wrong with
me. So . . . they wanted surgery. They talked about surgery. But I didn't
know what the surgery was going to be for, you know. However, the next

day, they put the stent in, and it immediately opened that bile duct. And that's when they found that I had a tumor pressing on the pancreas, which was pressing on the bile duct and closing it up. So I came home, I think the next day, and then I went to see a wonderful surgeon. And they thought that I should have this operation. But I didn't know what I was being operated on for, you know. I said, 'Well what are we being operated on for? Don't we have to make some kind of a diagnosis?' So they . . . then I decided to have laparoscopic diagnostic surgery [a less invasive type of surgery]. They did that and they actually did find the tumor, but they couldn't find any cancer cells. So I wasn't going to be operated on unless they could really tell me what was wrong. So I went, and then two months later I had to have another endoscopy [a procedure where a small tube is inserted into the gastrointestinal tract to visualize it] to put another stent in. And in April, no it was in June, after my third endoscopy, is when they found the cancer cells. And that's when they could prescribe some treatment for me. And we did . . . decide on surgery. And that was going to be in August."

I marvel at her manner of weaving together months of experience with the health care system, hospitalization, surgery, and subsequent procedures. She conveys the process with personal detail and clinical accuracy.

Mrs. Eck delves into the preoperative testing: "And I went through all kinds of pretesting, stress test, echocardiograms, carotid artery [angiography], CAT scans, MRIs, arteriogram. It was just go, go, go, go, go, you know, I was on the move practically all the time, from actually February and until I decided that I would have the surgery. The doctor said we have three choices. You can do nothing, you can join an experimental program, or you can have surgery. And then I said I think I'll elect the surgery. And doctor, the one doctor I went to at Stein, who suggested the surgery, I liked him very much. He was very nice. But I didn't feel really confident about it. You know, I just felt that, 'cause he'd say things like, 'Well if something happens on the table, we're not going to wake you up to tell you about it.' And you know, I just didn't feel comfortable with that. So that's when I decided to go to DeHaven. And then I had met with the oncology director, Dr. Clergery.[2] And that's when he said that we like to know what we're looking for, what it is we'd be operating for, we would like to really have a diagnosis. So that's when I had the different CAT scans and all that kind of thing. And then they sent me to the surgeon. And he explained to me the different options, and he said, 'If you want to live to be ninety, I think surgery is your best bet.' So that's OK with me. And I felt confident with him because he said he had done at least twenty-five of this type of surgery, in people in their eighties. And he had one patient, ninety-two, who still drove her own car in to see him. So I felt really, pretty confident about him, even though I knew it was a really major, major surgery. So I did all the pretesting. And we were scheduled to operate October, uh, August 22. And that Friday before the Sunday, they called me and said to be in the hospital Sunday at eleven o'clock. It wasn't ten minutes later, I get a call from the surgeon saying, 'We've canceled the surgery, the arteriogram showed two arteries involved with the tumor on the pancreas.' And he said, 'I wouldn't be able to get it all,' and he said, 'You wouldn't want me in there then,' you know. And he said, 'We need those arteries.' So, that canceled that. So then I went and they sent me to the doctor that gave us the radiation. So we decided on [a] twenty-eight [treatment] series of radiation, and five of chemotherapy. So I did that all of October, into September, all of October. And I went through fine, no problems really. And two days after I finished, I got radiation sickness." She laughs, less ruefully that I expect. "I was two weeks sick with that, you know."

Mrs. Eck goes on—not one to shy from vivid description or from her memory: "No appetite, couldn't eat anything, throwing up all the time. And it passed. And then I went back and they told me, you know, just I could eat anything I wanted. And they wanted me to eat. That was important. And that I'd get my taste buds back, and that I'd regain my appetite at some time along the line, you know. So at the end of all that, after a month, the doctor saw me again, and he said he didn't want to see me for three months, that my CAT scan was much improved over the other one, it had shrunk, the tumor had shrunk, and they were encouraged about that. Then I had to have my stent replaced. So this was now the fifth time I've been in for the stent. Every two months I had to do that. And that's an endoscopy every time. So I had that done, the twenty-second of November. And then, now I probably, I'll have to have it done in January, the end of January. But I don't see any of the other doctors till February—February and March." Mrs. Eck trails off and then returns to where she began her story. "So, and of course the hip is on the back burner."

Mrs. Eck begins again, refocusing her story on her life at home. After almost clinical details of nearly a year of sickness, uncertainty, and intervention, she returns to home and family.

"When I was in the hospital when they said I was yellow, and the doctor said, 'You're going to put your hip on the back burner.' So that's, I'm just dealing with that, you know. I use a cane, I use a walker. . . . And I have a wheelchair. And the girls take me out in the wheelchair, up and down the street, or around the block. And I even went shopping two times. So that was good."

But Mrs. Eck is ever mindful of the past year: "So it's just been, it's constant. One thing after another since last April, a year ago. . . ."

There is a brief lull in our conversation and Mrs. Eck offers a summary of her situation: "But all the while, I've had no pain, except with the hip. That's the only pain I've had. And I've had no pain with this pancreas thing. And I take Pancrease® [replacement pancreatic enzymes to help with digestion] before meals, and I take Darvocet® for what pain I have, and it works out OK. I sleep pretty good, and I'm happy, very happy, that I'm still here. Because in the very beginning, right after they thought I have the blocked bile duct, my daughter came in, the one that's the nurse, and she says, 'Mom,' she says, 'is there anything that you want to do? Or is there any place you want to go?' And I thought, whew, that's serious, you know. And I said, 'No, there isn't anything special I want to do, except go home and clean up my desk, and get my income tax stuff ready.' So [We both laugh.], that's what I did."

Mrs. Eck goes on and reveals her profound sense of family—husband, children, grandchildren all figure into her view of the world at this time: "And, and I know that they were all very concerned. Because they were here all the time, and everybody was bringing things in, and they were all doing things and all. So I know that it was something serious. But I wasn't going to get myself just in a terrible turmoil about it. Because I thought, I'm going to take this a day at a time, and what comes, what comes, and what is, is. So that's the way I've approached it. And I know when the doctor told me that my CAT scan looked a lot better I said, 'I'm happy.' You know. And I had a nice Christmas, you know, and managed to go out to dinner on my birthday."

I cannot help remarking that this is "wonderful." Mrs. Eck replies, "That was the first time I had really been out to dinner in a year." And I wonder aloud how she felt about it.

"It felt nice, but I, you know, they [restaurants] always give you so much, it's overwhelming. And, so I ate a little bit, you know. But it was good to be out. So that's really my story." She laughs softly.

I reflect to her what I hear in her story, telling her I had a sense that she was focused on living her life. She agrees: "I was going to just live each day as it came, and I never questioned the, you know, about what they said about how long I had. I always sensed that they knew, that they thought it was going to be about six months [to live]. The way they all acted and everything, I just felt, I have probably about six months. And . . . but I didn't think about that, I just put that aside. And I just thought I needed to go through all this, and see what the results are. So my tumor has shrunk. The only problem with it is, is that it also shrank the tissue around where the stent is. So when Dr. Trevelyan did the last stent he had trouble—trouble getting the plastic stent in. So he said we have to talk about this. And the surgeon, when I first talked to him about a permanent type stent, he said, 'Absolutely not.' He said, 'You'll have more trouble than you're in now.' So I told Dr. Trevelyan that, but now this time, and he said we have to do something about it. I asked Dr. Meister, he said OK. So I'm going to have a more permanent, a metal stent put in. Now every time I have a CAT scan, or an MRI, they ask me if I have any metal in my chest." We exchange information about what imaging can be used with metal devices in the body and which cannot. I tell her that you can generally have CAT scans, but that because MRI uses a magnet there can be some challenges.

Mrs. Eck confirms that this information is congruent with what she knows, and she continues: "Right. So at the end of January I'm going to have probably a metal stent put in. And I don't know how long that lasts, but it probably lasts a lot longer than this one does. Yes, because I think this, this I think would be my fifth stent."

I say, "That's a lot of endoscopies," and hear Mrs. Eck frame that repetitive procedure in her experience of knowing when her body needed it: "Yes. And when you come to a, near the end of it, you start getting itchy again. Then you know, when you start itching, it's time, yes."

Then Mrs. Eck thinks back to the first time she faced this problem: "But I had no idea. In January I had no idea that that itching really was anything. You know, I just thought they'd do some cleaning or something, you know. And when my daughter said, 'You look yellow,' and then I, when I was in the hospital, I had so many people coming in, I didn't know who they all were. And the . . . then the doctor came in, and she said, 'How do you think you look?' And I said, 'I think I look great.' I said, 'How do you think I look?' She said, 'I think you look yellow' [we both laugh at this]. Right. So it all cleared up and my eyes cleared up. Because I'll tell you, when I was in Stein Hospital, I . . . . they were so flattering to me. I said, I didn't want to leave, they were just—'You look so young for your age,' and 'Somebody made a mistake.' And the girls that came in to look at my eyes—'You have beautiful blue eyes,' you know. I said, boy, I don't want to leave this place." We both laugh again.

I am fascinated by this element of her story as it highlights the way in which age and appearance are inextricably intertwined in our social imaginations of what it is to be old. I say, "It's funny, though, how people might accept something when they hear eighty-five, but then they meet you and it . . . it doesn't seem to match. The eighty-five seems old and, and, and fragile. And you don't give that appearance." Mrs. Eck had just had her birthday at the time she was admitted to Stein Hospital.

Mrs. Eck finds irony in her experience of hospitalization after we discuss age and social preconceptions of old age: "The other night, when I had, uh, what is it, the laparoscopic surgery, they did that at five o'clock in the afternoon, and I didn't get into a bed till eleven. I was in recovery, and the next morning at six o'clock this group of people [her medical team] comes in, and you know, I'm not even awake yet. And they come in, this one, the lead person leans over and he says [she raises her voice], 'You have to have surgery!' Just like that. And I just looked at him, and I didn't even answer him. I just said, 'I wouldn't have surgery in there if you paid me to have it.' So then the head doctor came in that night, and he said, 'What are you going to do?' And I said, 'I'm going home, and I'm going to mull it all over.' And that's what I did, I went home, I thought about it, and I said, 'I'm going to DeHaven. I'm going to get another opinion.'"

And I think to myself of the rather annoying and common habit that many people have of yelling at older people, believing all to be hard of hearing and yelling an effective solution. But instead of following this thought, I ask, "Have you always been that way? You know, just to take the time and . . . and say I'm going to make my own decisions, but I'm going to make them in my own time. Have you done that?" I want to confirm the commonly held idea that people maintain personal style and preferences through adulthood and into later life.

Mrs. Eck replies easily, "I think most likely I have, yes." We meditate on this idea a moment, exchanging small comments with one another as we look for the thread of meaning in the conversation that she wants to pick up and follow. She finds it quickly.

"Well you know I always say that we've lived through really trying times, our generation. I mean we had the Depression when I was pretty young, I think I was about twelve. And we had the war [World War II]. And my husband was in the war, he was a pilot. But, and then you knew that anything could happen, at any time. But you didn't dwell on it, you just didn't, you just took each day as it came and tried to get through it the best you can. And there always, during that time of the war we all did something. We ran too, you know, I was a nurse's aide in two hospitals."

Thinking of the trials that must have faced wives waiting for husbands to return from combat, I ask, "Were you and your husband married before you . . . ?"

"No, we were not married yet. I was here with my parents and my sister. And so I did that [worked as a nurse's aide], and I sold war bonds at the movies. And we could always, we did that for the first show, and then the second show we could go watch the movie. So that was always good. So there were things that I did. And we all did something. And we just did it, you know. If we didn't have meat or butter, or whatever, we lived without it, you know. We had to have stamps for gas, we had to have stamps for shoes, things like that. Everybody pulled together. There was no griping or anything. So I think that probably was good training for later on, when you raised a family and met problems, you know. So we had five kids, and they all turned out good. They all have good jobs and they, we all, we all raised likeable children. So we [she and her husband] think that's a good accomplishment. And they all have been just wonderful to me."

I remind Mrs. Eck that she had mentioned that one of her daughters visits her every morning to provide care and offer support now that her mother is less mobile due to her hip problem.

Mrs. Eck replies: "Yes, that's really very nice. I mean it really is, you know, I mean and they always write and they visit and they explain how much they love me, how much they enjoy doing what they're doing for me, and all those, you know. And I enjoy having them, you know. I know it's taken a lot of their time. And they don't want me to fall, that's the main thing. And so that's why they insist that I wait for somebody to bring me down and take me out. And I've said, 'I can do this myself, I don't need all this.' And I tried to tell them, 'Look I . . . I can do this myself.' But no, they all want to do it. And my husband, the same way. 'I'm your husband, and I—' [she laughs], you know, all this. So he pushes me up the steps at night. And, and I think it's, it's been nice, it really has been. I mean I think all the kids have gotten closer together too.

"They seemed scattered, you know. It's like my one daughter, Beth, lives in New Jersey. And Patrick lives in New York. And Joe lives in Vermont. Sue lives in New Jersey. And Tracy lives [nearby]. She's pretty much right around the corner from . . . yes. So she comes every morning. And some mornings, when Sue's not working, she comes. And then she may come down and tuck me in bed. And they have seemed to like that idea of tucking me in." We both laugh.

"They [all of her children] do, they have time with one another. Like Joe will cook tonight and my daughter Sue is coming for dinner. And my niece Mary Jo and my niece Gwen have both been very greatly supportive too. Mary Jo comes on Saturday mornings. They're my sister's children; my sister passed in 2002."

Mrs. Eck continues, shifting the course of her story to reminisce about her sister: "Yes, and we were just two sib—two sisters, no, no brothers or sisters. And we were, did everything together, we were almost like twins."

I ask the obvious question: "Were you close in age?"

"No, I was three years older," Mrs. Eck says. "But she was the one, the take-charge one. She took charge of everything, and she was always saying to me, 'I don't know how you do it. You always get everybody to do everything for you. You don't do anything, you've got everybody doing something for you.' So this summer, I'm sitting on the porch, and I'm doing something, and somebody said, 'I'll do this for you.' And I said, 'Uh-oh, there she is up there: "So there she is again! She's got somebody to do it for her!"' [She laughs.] She always killed me about it—'You can get people to do things for you.' So . . . I just, that day I said, oh my, she's up there saying, 'You did it again.' Oh!"

I remark, "But it's funny how we remember those things, and then, and how they, they're meaningful and funny at the same time."

And Mrs. Eck goes on, recalling memories of her sister: "It's a lifelong— She always, and I can remember my mother would, if something wasn't right at the store [the family business], when my sister and I, and I don't know whether she went with me to get it, but I had it and came home with it. And my mother would say, 'Now you just take this back, you know, get something, get something different.' And I'd always say to Jane, she'd come with me and I'd say, 'You go in. You go in and do it.'" She laughs. "And so she goes, she always bailed me out, all the time."

I probe gently, with a smile, "That's what little sisters are for?"

"I only had the one sister. So we were really very close. She lived just three blocks from me. So that, for the first, for six years after we were married we lived in [a town close by]. And, but then this was my mother and father's home, and my mother got sick, and my father wanted to have a smaller house. So he offered this house to my husband and me. And so we sold our first house and got, bought this one. And we had three children when we moved here. And then we had two after we got here. And it was, it's been great. It's been plenty of room for them. I never had to worry because they were always out in the backyard, playing, you know."

That memory trails into her marriage: "We've been married sixty-one years. And uh, we've just had a wonderful life, I mean it's just been great. We get along real good together, we're real friends, you know. And I knew my husband, I've met him about 19 . . . 1938. We were married in 1944. We were both in college. So it turned out just great."

I want to know more and ask, "Did you know in 1938 or did . . . did it take a while for you to know that he was the one?"

"You know I . . . I felt it the minute I saw him. He was so easy to talk to. He made you feel so comfortable, and it was funny how we met, because my cousin, he had picked my cousin up. They were going to have a party at Walt's home in [a nearby town]. And they had their basement all fixed up with a dance floor and a bar and all that. So they stopped at my house, and my cousin asked if I would like to go this party. So I asked my mother and my mother said no. And so I prevailed upon them and they let me go. And when I went up there, Walt was the bartender. And I sat on the stool facing him and he was just so comfortable to be with. And he brought me home that night. Then I didn't hear from him at all for a couple of weeks. So I thought well, you know, nothing's going to amount to that, you know. But then he called me, and we went out. And I just, I just, I just cared for him right from the beginning, you know. I don't know what he saw in me, but he called and called, so, but and we got along really well together. We always have, we always have. No big blow ups or anything. One or two . . . [We both laugh.] But he would always say to me, 'If you don't, if you don't blow your stack at least once a day, I wouldn't think it was you.' Because then I'd turn around, and he's sitting there with a big smile on his face and how could I be mad at somebody like that, you know, so, that's how we managed. And he's never really gotten mad at me. I've gotten mad a few times myself, because I had red hair. A bit of a temper, yes. So we had, out of our children we had three redheads. The boys both with heads red. And one girl was brunette, one was red, and one was blonde.

"Here's to good life. I mean we're both eighty-six now. My husband's birthday's December 15, and mine's December 30. So every year I tell him, you're a year older than I am, for two weeks.

"And, so we both feel blessed that we've had a happy life, good kids. So we can't ask for anything more than that. And we're both eighty-six. Then there's ninety, and happier still. [We both laugh.] So that's what I'm doing, I'm taking it a day at a time and fighting the battle."

I ask particularly about her choice of phrase: "And do you think of it as a battle?"

Mrs. Eck says, "I do think of it as a battle. [Each day] a little bit better or maybe a little bit, maybe someday it'll be a little worse, I don't know yet, you know. But for now, I feel good. Some days I don't feel as good as others but most days I feel good. So I really can't complain. I'm happy with, I'm happy with the treatments I've had, and I might have to have some more chemotherapy, they said, just to keep things on an even keel. And I don't mind that. So I just feel like I've, I feel like I've really done a good job this year. You know I, I've tried to maintain balance. I've tried to stay healthy and peppy, as much as I can be peppy with this, my bad hip that, you know, I don't get, I don't get dejected."

I ask, "Are there things that you do for yourself to . . . to keep your outlook that way?"

"I love to read. And that's really most of my pastime now, is to read. And, and I don't, I'm just not depressed, just not depressed about it. But I was very shocked. I have to admit to that. That I never, ever thought that would happen to me, that I would have cancer, never. In fact I used to say to myself, well that'll never happen to me 'cause we don't have that in our family. And we don't, we don't have any of that in our family. And, but that was a big shock to me."

I wonder aloud how she understands it, noting that I think many people would share her reaction. Mrs. Eck replies: "Yes. I . . . I . . . I just couldn't believe it, I really, I just went, 'This can't be happening to me.' I thought I'd die of a heart attack or something, 'cause that's what, my family all heart problems. And my sister died of a heart attack. And I never, I just never let that into my thoughts, you know. And even, even in the beginning when we really didn't know for sure that this was a . . . cancer, I knew I had a tumor, but I didn't know whether it was a benign tumor. And even if it was a benign tumor it was causing a lot of trouble. So either way, it was probably going to do its damage. But I just, I . . . I think I faced it, I faced the fact that I knew that maybe I could go, you know, in six months. And [she laughs] I did smile though because my, when I was in the hospital, before I went to Stein, and I overheard the conversation about this, 'She might die on the table,' and then they was . . . they were saying, 'Mother do you want to go anywhere? Is there anything you want to do?' and all this, I thought, can't be having much time here. So the one night my one daughter came in, the other daughter that comes and helps me. She says, 'Now, Mother, what do you want to do with this?' You know, 'What do you want to do with your jewelry?' You know, do you want to give this, any special piece to different ones? She got the notepaper out, and writing, you know. And I have two sets of trains, and, 'Well now what do you want to do about your trains?' You know. And my little granddaughter, who's ten years old, was sitting there. And I said to her, 'I want to give'—I have two granddaughters—I said, 'I want to give my trains, one to each granddaughter.' One's an old gas train, and one's a newer-model gas train. And the little one says, 'I'll take the old one.' The ten-year-old says, 'I'll take the old one.' [We both laugh.] So, I said I haven't given them to them yet. [But] they're scheduled to get them." She laughs again.

I remark that she is well past the six-month prognosis she was originally given. "Yes. Almost a year, coming up on it. . . . But I didn't let it get me down. 'Cause I just said, no, I'm going to take this one day at a time. I'm going to try to get up every day and see what the day brings, you know. But I've been busy. I have been busy, because we've just been on the go, going to all those appointments and all these tests, and all, and I also had my hip injected in June. It helped for a while. And I can't have that done again. But I had to go under anesthesia for that, just a regular surgery, and I almost, and I've had five endoscopies, and the other thing, they poke the holes in you, I always forget the name of that, the laparoscopic surgery. And then with all the CAT scans and the, everything, and all the blood tests, I've been busy. . . . And this summer I got to the beach four times. I couldn't walk to the beach, but they, they, the municipality has wheelchairs, with the big tires on them—that go on the sand. So they wheeled me to the beach four times, and that was really nice. You know, so I think I've had a, kind of an exciting year. Yes. And every day we went for radiation I had to be at DeHaven at quarter of ten every morning. So we had to leave here by nine o'clock, you know, to get out there. So it was, you know, keeping you on the move. Get up, get the shower, get dressed, get out, you know? Yes. And that's another thing, they [her daughters] help me with my shower, because it's hard for me to get in the tub [because of her hip]. So getting my leg, so they come down and do that, which, I get out and get in, right, you know. So that's, that's pretty much been my year."

I begin to close by asking if she has any plans. Mrs. Eck replies, "I'm going to the shore [the southern New Jersey coast] next week for the week. Yes, we're going to go down Sunday. And I have a place at the shore, so we're going down, stay the week. And then I'll be due for a stent change, and back to the doctors. And maybe I'll have to have the chemotherapy, I don't know yet. So, but outside of that, there's no place I really want to go. I've been a lot, to a lot of places. I've been to many places overseas, and I'm not interested in going back. I don't want to go on an airplane again, after having that pneumonia. Then I had it two years later, the same thing. And I . . . I enjoy my home. I really, I really do. And I don't feel lonely. I mean, they come in the morning and I'm really set up in the meantime. Sometimes they make my lunch for me. Sometimes I go out and get it myself. And they leave. Watch some TV. I like to watch the news. And I like to watch the cooking shows. And I never did cook. [We both laugh.] I used to cook. I . . . I don't do the cooking anymore. And I don't think I'd probably ever make what they make, but I like to watch them. You know, something different. And then as soon as, as soon as they put an ingredient in that I say, 'Oh, I don't like that,' that's it. That's that, forget that, forget that recipe. [We both laugh.] Yes, that's really that, and then Walt gets home at five-thirty. So we just have dinner, maybe about six-thirty. Watch the news together."

We talk for a few minutes about a mine collapse in West Virginia that has been in the news, a tragedy with only one miner surviving, and Mrs. Eck picks up our exchange about the fragile nature of life and says: "[Life] . . . it absolutely changes. It's, I told you my sister died in 2002, and it was on Thanksgiving Day. And we always have Thanksgiving together. And she was here, she cooked the turkey, did all the vegetables. I did . . . I did . . . I always made the pies. So I was making the pies, she was getting the vegetables and all things ready the day before. And then on Thanksgiving Day she brought the turkey up from the basement to the refrigerator, start that readying in the oven and all. We had Thanksgiving dinner. And she lives, she lived with me in the, in the wintertime. She came up at Thanksgiving to stay the winter, because she lived at the shore and it was so quiet and alone down there. So she came on a Tuesday, and then Thursday was Thanksgiving. We got through dinner and everything and about nine-thirty she said she was going to her daughter's home for the night. And it used to be her home. So her daughter, Mary

Jo, was with her, and she came over. I was sitting in that chair and she came over and she said, 'I'll pick you up for the hairdresser's at ten-thirty tomorrow morning.' That's, we said goodnight to each other, and I went to bed about eleven-thirty. And our phone rang around one o'clock in the morning. And my daughter, the one that's the nurse, said, 'Go downstairs and open the door, and go back to bed.' And I thought, what is that all about? So I came up and I said to my husband, 'Sue just called and she said go down and open the door and go get back in bed.' So a few minutes later she came. And she started, 'Now you know, Mom, you know Aunt Jane hasn't been well, and she's had these heart problems.' And I jumped out of bed and I said, 'You mean she's dead?' And she said yes. And I looked up. She [her sister] had gone, her daughter was going up to bed, and Jane [her sister] went up about eleven-thirty, talked to Mary Jo, in her room, went in the bathroom, they all heard the water running and all. And came back into her room, took her sneaks off and all and had her pajamas in her hand, fell over dead. Yes. Mary Jo just heard a little noise, and she went in, called 911 and all. Yes, so that was a horrible shock for everybody. Yes. So this year they didn't want to do Thanksgiving like we always did. 'Cause the little kids were just so disturbed by all these things happening, you know. My daughter's sister-in-law lost her husband two . . . two Thanksgivings ago. So they were two in a row. One, one year, and one the next. So this year we tried to do it differently. And we just, I forget what we did [laughter], we just, we had the turkey and all but . . . We had it kind of buffet style, you know, where we didn't sit at the table. Right. So it's been eventful. Yes. It's been, I can't say it's been a bad year this year. You know."

Mrs. Eck returns to her current experience of daily life: "And I found everybody to be so nice. Everybody I came in contact with, no matter who it was, they were all so nice. Patients, you know, they'd see you sitting there, and they'd be waiting for a ride or something in there, and they'd always speak, 'And are you going home?' You know, no, I'm just coming, you know, or something like that. And then they'd tell you about what they were, went through. And, 'Did you lose your hair?' No, I didn't lose my hair. 'Well I lost my hair.' And I said to the one woman, 'Well your hair looks really very nice.' And she, 'Well it's a wig.' [We both laugh.] I said, 'Well it's very flattering.' But they all, just, and some of them [other patients] are so much worse than you are, you know? But they were so, so good. Well after you finish your therapy, you ring the bell. They have a bell on a flap, and you go out and you ring the bell, you know. And people stay in the room and all clap and all, you know. So it's, it's been a good year. And all the people, some of them are really very sick, but they, they carry it off well. They don't try to burden everybody else with it. And I think that's nice. So we all feel like we're in the battle together.

And we're all doing, taking it one day at a time, you know. It's what you have to do. . . . 'Cause there's too many other things to live for, you know, I mean there's interesting things to do, you know. My husband always says, 'If I can get up and put my two feet on the floor in the morning I'm good for the day.' So . . . [She laughs.] So that's pretty much my experience for the year."

I tell her, "It's a really good story," and she replies, "I hope it helps somebody else." She goes on to make another connection: "And you know, even my roommates that I had in the hospital, I've become really very good friends with them. I mean when I had my pneumonia I was in for three weeks. So my roommate was in for the same amount of time almost. And we became such good friends, we were on the phone to each other, talking for like an hour at a time. And then this last time, my roommate has called me. I was only in the hospital five days there, but she calls me and wants to know how I am and all, you know. I know I haven't, I haven't gone over to DeHaven once, I've met someone that wasn't nice. I mean everybody is. And I do enjoy, and you know it's just car after car after car going in there. It's amazing, it's amazing to see the number of people. That . . . that was an eye opener for me. You know. But everybody's doing what they have to do. And it's, and they're all smiling. . . . We go for the labs [blood drawn for laboratory tests], you have to sign in, and then the one woman that kind of directs you, she, once she said, 'Do you need a hot blanket?' And every time I would go, she would go get a hot blanket and wrap me up in it, you know. One day I think I had three hot blankets on. I mean they just do things that are so nice for you, you know. Makes you feel good. It does, it does. You know, and like one day I had ten, I also had blood taken out. And I always have a hard time, they have a hard time finding my veins. But they all do it swiftly and accurately that it's not that bad, you know. But I said, no wonder it's hard to find, you've taken it all out of there. [We both laugh.] I know, I know. Well I guess, growing up we probably thought it was really as old as [that], if you ever got to be eighty. And I just don't feel it, you know? And I don't think I act it. And I'm happy. [We both laugh.] And we've been blessed, because my husband's in pretty good health, and you know, I'm, I've been in good health up to this time. I've had excellent health. And that's, that was a big shock to me, was the fact that, you know . . ."

I fill in: "You never expected it?"

Mrs. Eck replies: "No, never expected it. I was really happy, I'm, we, we're really blessed, we say that we're really blessed. Whatever happens, we've been blessed. God has been good to us. My daughter Tracy is the one that runs our store now. And my daughter Sue is the nurse. She's been a nurse for thirty-some years, she graduated in 1970. She's an emergency room nurse. And my daughter Beth is our middle daughter, and she's the one who lives in Hopewell, so she comes when she can. I have, she's, she always spends the day after Christmas here, they're here Christmas night, and she's wonderful the next day, because she cleans up after all the open packages, you know. We came, we went to my niece's for Christmas dinner, and we came back here and opened packages. And everybody, so it was wall-to-wall paper, you know."

Mrs. Eck ended her story with the Christmas just past. The blessings of her family—her own children and those of her beloved sister—were seemingly laid before us for our mutual contemplation. I am touched by how Mrs. Eck tells of prevailing over cancer and—with even greater challenge—a health care system apparently ill prepared to ease her journey through it. Mrs. Eck's contemplation of blessings among the battles of cancer and cancer treatment takes a humorous turn as we both resist closing our time together. Mrs. Eck tells me a charming story about how she and Mr. Eck are known by family, neighbors, and even some of their children's acquaintances for their standing Wednesday lunch date. For years, she tells me after my tape recorder has been turned off, she and her husband shared a private ritual. They would have lunch, the same lunch, every Wednesday afternoon. They savored hot dogs, nothing special mind you, Mrs. Eck exclaimed, just hot dogs, washed down with champagne. While her radiation side effects have resolved and she is eating again at the time we meet, Mrs. Eck notes wistfully that her taste for champagne has not returned. She wants very much to enjoy Wednesday lunch of champagne and hot dogs with her husband once again.

I left Mrs. Eck that afternoon, compelled by the image of her private lunch with her husband of many years. Champagne and hot dogs—it is a menu I think of being simultaneously romantic and youthful. Somehow hot dogs, with all their connotations of summer cookouts, young children, and family holidays, are the inexpensive sandwich of young couples who might not be able to afford much. Put hot dogs together with champagne as Mrs. Eck and her husband did for their standing date and you have a quirky combination that becomes a shared and private ritual. This story captivated me the most of all those that Mrs. Eck told me that January day, because, as a nurse, I love knowing what makes the people who become my patients—or in this case, the object of my contemplation—the people they are at the time I know them. In Mrs. Eck's story, champagne and hot dogs for Wednesday lunch with her husband became emblematic of who she was as daughter, wife, sister, mother, and aunt and what she valued as she wove together her biography for me. Mrs. Eck's pancreatic cancer shifted from its prominence when we first began her story to its place among several challenges she had faced in her life. She spoke most movingly of her relationships with her family and of her sorrow at her sister's sudden death. Her battle against pancreatic cancer seemed far more about maintaining her perception of self and her life as she knew it. Surmounting cancer in cure was not in the mix of concerns that Mrs. Eck addressed with me. Maintaining her life as she wished it against the mundane battles of radiologic scans, radiation therapy, and the stents that helped her avoid jaundice took center stage. Mrs. Eck left me with a profound sense that she felt blessed by life, family, and faith despite the battles she faced against her cancer and the inherent challenges in treating it.

Chapter 2
Being Old, Having Cancer

Current social meaning associated with being old and having cancer maintains a tension between culturally embedded impressions of this state of being and the reality of its demography and individual experience. The societal impression of what it is to be old and have cancer is, in the largest and most abstract sense, one of despair, suffering, and death. The topic of aging and cancer generally elicits responses that distance the listener from perceived specters of debility, despair, and death. Yet the demographics of cancer in American society and the stories of older people and their families point to a far different reality.

Mrs. Eck's story, centered as it is in family, is at once uniquely her own and belonging to the American woman of her generation, from her ties to the home in which she grew up and raised her own family to her physical presence of grace, care, and warmth. She tells a story that transcends her gender as much as it is couched in her life place as daughter, sister, wife, mother, and aunt. The balance between the battles of cancer and particularly cancer treatment and the blessings of her unique and particular life mostly lived are Mrs. Eck's alone. It is her personal story of living her life in the face of a cancer that is characterized both medically and socially as life closing. Mrs. Eck does not really portray her life as closed, however, and has desires and dreams that frame a future she desires. True, her cancer and the treatment it entails hamper that future. Mrs. Eck's future includes a return to her Wednesday lunch of champagne and hot dogs with her husband to whom she is clearly and quietly devoted.

Mrs. Eck's story reminds me of countless other stories I have heard from old people—my patients, my relatives, my friends, colleagues' family members, even acquaintances. Few offer as sweet a symbol of sustaining relationship as does a shared lunch of champagne and hot dogs. Some use the language of battle more painfully. Others do not speak of blessings, recalling loss more often than triumph. But all the people who are older and have cancer who have told me their stories in part or as a whole are always singularly themselves.

The battles of cancer are trying—whether they are told as such and whether they include confrontations such as when Mrs. Eck heard her own life-threatening prognosis baldly pronounced within her earshot. The older people I have treated commonly speak directly of the battles against cancer as disease and those of cancer treatment. They also speak of the experiences of feeling and being ill with the symptoms of cancer and of other diseases, such as Mrs. Eck's hip problem. And they tell of battles with a health care system ill equipped in both human and technological terms to integrate the complex care they need to manage life with cancer, in addition to other diseases, and of possibly already limited physical function and sometimes mental capacity. Importantly, these battles exist temporally in a far larger scope of their lives—with their earlier battles won or lost—lives that are mostly lived.

These lives are made intricate by the experiences of decades lived and the desires, fears, and needs in what lies ahead. They are lives generally not given over easily to cancer, its treatment, or its prognosis. While the youthful social metric for cancer is full engagement in a singular war, the older people I have met, treated, and studied present an image of battles on many fronts, recalibrated success, and the wisdom of decades braved and years anticipated. I have rarely found the stereotype of being old and having cancer—enveloping debility, endless despair, and proximate death—borne out in the stories I have heard from those who are considered old and who have or have had cancer. This is not to say that being old and having cancer never debilitates those older people who are affected—it most certainly can—or that it does not provoke despair—it often does for people of any age—or that older people do not die of cancer—they do at rates second only to cardiovascular disease. Rather, my argument is that the monochromatic stereotype is, in my experience, far from the reality I have observed over the course of two decades.

I often speak publicly on being old and having cancer. I speak to professional groups about care for older people who have cancer. I speak to lay audiences about cancer and caring for themselves or—if the audience is younger—an older friend or relative with cancer. I generally ask these audiences to consider their own lives in relation to being old and having cancer. Many in the audience, whether old or young, can immediately identify someone they know and love as fitting a socially bound image of being old and having cancer—around sixty years of age or older, living with cancer or having lived through it—these are real people living real lives. Knowing or loving someone who is old and has cancer is an increasingly common experience in American families. But these people do not become their cancers, as pervasive understandings would have us believe. In fact, these older people often fight against such an appellation by the health care system and clinicians who treat them as though they have nothing in their lives but cancer treatment and other conditions. They may also battle two distinct social reactions, directed at them by people who are generally not close enough to know them well but are close enough to know they have cancer. First, older adults are often the recipients of distant and well-meaning, stereotypical pity—"Oh, how sad! Are you on hospice care?"—which presumes that the cancer is immediately lethal, which it may well not be. This pity may, however, reinforce long-held understandings of older adults who remember cancer from their younger years as fatal, isolating, and untreatable—all of which are untrue today. Second are the mean-spirited, judgmental questions conveying blame for a lifestyle that supposedly resulted in cancer. Questions may be as blunt as "So, did you smoke?" even when the cancer is not linked to tobacco use, or as numbing as "What did you do to get that cancer?" calling up the decades-old construction of cancer as a disease of personal responsibility. Juxtaposing the image of debility, despair, and death and the responses such a stereotype generates against the lives and relationships that characterize the daily life of older people highlights how incommensurate the socially proscribed impression of being old and having cancer is with the daily lives lived by those individuals. How then are the socially constructed, largely negative images maintained in the face of contravening daily experience?

"What is it to be old and have cancer in our society?" is a multifarious question that has long held my interest. The intricacies of late life and chronic, sometimes life-threatening disease have been revealed to me in the stories of patients for whom I provide care, in conversation with the participants met in research projects, and in the impressions on families attending public lectures on elder or cancer care. These stories, told in many contexts, for many listeners, and by many tellers, beget equally detailed and nuanced depictions of the state of being old and having cancer. Immediate personal impressions for the older person and those close to him or her are likely colored by intimate details and significant connections.

Cancer experienced by an individual as a personal disease is colored by that individual's history. Life lived is recalled in memories of earlier times, other illnesses survived, obstacles faced, and losses endured. But the experience of cancer may recede somewhat in the face of other activities—pleasant or challenging—that shape daily life unless or until that daily life is confronted or overwhelmed by the effects of the cancer and its treatment. Cancer may not stand front and center, for example, in the life of an older person who has other chronic diseases such as painful arthritis or who has responsibilities in caring for others such as grandchildren or an ill spouse or sibling. Far different ideas emerge if one thinks about an older individual one knows who is living with cancer rather than if one questions what it means to be old and have cancer. Social and cultural meaning bound what it means to be old and have cancer. Shared images of growing old and being ill, common conceptions of cancer and cancer treatment, and other losses attached to aging, illness, and ability percolate through society. Those images permeate distanced understandings of being old and having cancer unless they are countered by personal knowledge of more immediate stories and narratives directly told.

The sociocultural history of aging in our society is complex and not easily reversed. Centrally, themes of the moral and immoral impinge upon behavior and ideals of success in late life. The idea of living well, meaning morally within a largely Protestant Christian frame congruent with the primary force of postcolonial American culture, creates a transcendent, persistent image of late life (Cole 1992; Leichter 2003). The successful—that is, moral—aging person is one who is independent and yet serves as a beacon of morality and right living for subsequent generations. Independence is perhaps nothing more than the absence of inwardly and outwardly perceived burden in attendant loss of function. Near obsession with physical health and fitness imbues modern interpretations of anticipated functional loss in late life. Such obsession suggests that the successful older adult must strive achieve almost superhuman images of physical fitness and implied notions of necessary mental fitness. This transcendent image is one without debility and disease and encompasses an often beatific physicality of the kindly old person with snowy hair and beneficent demeanor.

Disease and illness are understood to jeopardize fitness at any age, and especially in late life. Such a danger may be perceived as far more threatening than the resultant physical reality. Old age connotes a fragility that intertwines myriad threads of social and cultural apprehension with the tangible effects of aging. In the past, disease often directly implied receding moral character before biomedicine and the defense of genetic and similarly fixed antecedents. Now the implication is far less direct and more deeply intertwined with historically mediated sociocultural effects. In the past, contracting disease was often laced with moral overtones of weakness and hapless or even evil behavior. These implications even survive today: consider current images of those who smoke tobacco and are diagnosed with lung or other cancers. Even the language of disease— one *contracts* a disease—connotes behavioral complicity. Those who live life immorally endure the physical ills that represent the opposite image of transcendent moral spirit and fit physical being within a Protestant notion of aging and late life (Cole 1992).

Cancer exemplifies moral entailment of behavior and uncertainty in disease. No illustration of such entangled social thought is more compelling than contemporary rhetoric around tobacco consumption and cancer. The story of tobacco and cancer accretes political overtones day by day. Paradoxically, lung cancer is the disease that vilifies those who use tobacco, and yet not all lung cancer can be linked to tobacco consumption. Not all those who use tobacco develop lung cancer, though popular impressions contravene this clinical fact. Patients who have lung cancer but never smoked may complain of the tiring litany of blaming questions about tobacco and other malefic behavior. Is lung cancer a socially obvious cancer because of associations with smoking, perceptions of poor prognosis or some other characteristic?

Yet cancer, morality, aging, and debility thread strikingly through the fabric of American social history. Patterson outlines the prurient intersection of disgust and fear triggered by cancer in America (Patterson 1987). Until recent decades, cancer compelled aversive interest as it transformed lives and created suffering. Families attempted to manage a generally deadly disease in any way possible, relying on limited medical care and facing extreme nursing need.

My first reading of *The Dread Disease: Cancer and Modern American Culture* (Patterson 1987) more than twenty years ago revealed the story of Ulysses S. Grant, declining and impoverished after his presidency. Grant struggled to provide for his family as he suffered the effects of throat cancer as a man in his sixth decade. The mental image of Grant sitting on his porch, feverishly writing what would become his best-selling memoir of the Civil War, impelled me toward an understanding of aging and cancer framed by sociocultural implications of aging and disease joined with historically themed images of being old and having cancer.

The dominant image of physical ills in late life associated with European Protestant Christian understandings of self, life, and aging holds undeniable social powers of judgment and exclusion (Cole 1992). Though the hold is certainly weaker than it was in colonial or even Victorian American times—with the rather romantic view of tuberculosis, or consumption—the sway of personal blame and just punishment in disease and dysfunction remains evident today (Cole 1992; Leichter 2003). Social discourse on prevention of cancer, as well as rhetoric around HIV infection—with behavioral risks couched in choice and judgment—and type 2 diabetes—with ever more explicit connections drawn to body weight and the obesity epidemic, make personal responsibility and consequences the overarching theme of common dialogue. Such dialogue testifies to contemporary perceptions of behavior and fitness in understanding health and disease. Those who face such disease are, broadly speaking, seen as singularly culpable despite mitigating influences of fixed risk, complex social forces, and factors that impinge on behavior and risk modification (Leichter 2003).

Beyond social exclusion, this rather punitive power discriminates as a received view of what meaning being old and ill holds in our society. Perspectives originating in cultures outside the Anglo-European realm recede against the backdrop of morally charged, personally responsible, inevitably individual understandings of being old and having cancer (Leichter 2003; Cole 1992). Emphasis on the individual and autonomous character opposes other cultural impressions of self and even the daily experience of actions and relationships through life. Biomedical notions of disease and illness implicate behavioral effects in cellular processes—an intellectual leap for most, taken on faith in biomedicine and allopathic treatment. Discomfort with the idea of aging as inevitable engenders a sense that old age can be made diseaselike and thus approached in the same manner applied to cancer and other diseases. Despite cellular and subcellular knowledge, fixed risk, and ineluctable consequences of being human, aging—like these diseases—can be denied and, barring that, modified. Biomedicine, as the means through which the dominant European American Protestant Christian understandings of self, life, and aging seem often enacted, then surmounts other sociocultural understandings of aging and disease. This received view is rendered in myriad messages throughout society, subordinating understandings of self that extend beyond the individual, of life beyond the biological, and of aging beyond multifaceted loss.

Rapidly advancing knowledge and technology in biomedicine complicates the nature, perception, and understanding of being old and having a disease like cancer. In the past, slow-evolving influences situated such human phenomena so that we could grasp its salience to daily life. Over the course of the twentieth century, for example, life expectancy moved from the fifth to the eighth decade of life through slow improvements in health and social care. Watershed discoveries such as pasteurization and penicillin emerged at a pace where change could be assimilated. Increasingly, society is pelted by discoveries and changes that shift understandings of any number of phenomena. Discovery and change in aging and cancer typify this shift. Daily media coverage of scientific and medical discoveries bombards professional and lay audiences alike with evanescent messages of antiaging and cancer prevention. Fast-moving bullets impress notions of evading the inevitable through right living and ageless fitness. Images and values of health and social care, especially care for the aged, then shift whether or not their actual practice changes. These imagined and tangible experiences and understandings collide on both social and personal levels. They inevitably alter the experiences of individuals and families. Living in our society implies some exposure, impossible to avoid altogether, to socially shared and exchanged understandings. What was understood as true of health, disease, and care yesterday may be questioned or disputed tomorrow, shaking confidence and surety. Attached meaning is drawn into question. Accordingly, meaning attached to being old and having cancer fragments or blurs in the face of rapidly advancing knowledge and technology in the areas of aging and oncology.

No one can avoid the penetrating and repetitive but also evocative societal messages that shape the impressions, and indeed the experience, of the state of being old. Consider the pervasive nature of age in our society. Germane or not, chronological age shows itself everywhere in social discourse. Celebrating birthdays, creating profiles for identification, and outlining family history come up as useful, relevant considerations of chronological age. Judging mental capacity, arbitrating social desirability, and delimiting physical fitness are too frequently attached to chronological age. Chronological age may exclude individuals from access to services or activities. While trends in politically correct language and action make overt exclusion difficult, self-exclusion or self-stereotyping— the incorporation of social messages—may achieve similar elision.

In a society struck by normative visual characteristics of human form and function, characteristic features in images of being old are inextricable from judging chronological age. Many adults whose physical presence connotes a certain perceived age can tell manifold stories of exclusion and derision. The woman who carefully counts her change in a grocery store but looks young will irritate and may be confronted, but only as an equal sparring partner. The woman who carefully counts her change and looks old and frail more likely elicits silent frustration, palpable pity, eye-rolling derision, or contemptuous epithets. Age makes the difference here and in innumerable situations we face in our daily lives. In fact, behaviors that overturn these socially mediated constructions of what it is to be old are remarkable, capturing attention as unexpected and unusual.

More overtly, mental capacity and memory are made pathologically worrisome by old age. A young man who forgets occasional appointments, names, or words is considered overworked, overscheduled, and "stressed out." A man old enough to qualify for Medicare who forgets the same occasional items evokes concerns of disease—Alzheimer's disease imbues the current American consciousness with paradigmatic fears of losing one's mind—while consideration of work and schedule recedes into nothingness. The intersection of abstract notions of old age and the state of being old then seems tied to that which is visually apprehended to connote being old and being ill.

Behaviors contradicting socially mediated constructions of what it is to be old garner specific attention. These behaviors must illustrate positive impressions of physical or mental function that exceed expectations of cumulative loss and social desynchrony or overt withdrawal. Successful aging, as it is linguistically juxtaposed against usual—that is, typical aging—allegorizes such contradictory behavior. The language of successful aging opposes usual aging in gerontology, embedded as it is in the conceptual language of the discipline. Rowe and Kahn (1987) are among the most prominent proponents of this perspective, as they argued for understanding aging in function, functional decline, and capacity for improvement in the late 1980s. Successful aging permeates the nature of scientifically oriented clinical inquiry and reasoning in gerontology. Hazzard's (1997) clarion voice speaks for many who envision the future of gerontology as equating the usual with the successful. While the dominance of successful aging offers confirming images of being old, it excludes positively constructed impressions for those who cannot or do not fulfill the ideal of success. We leave little room for the very real and multifaceted heterogeneity of late life.

Idealization of a functionally mediated image of being old and the impression of aging lacks a constructive place for what lies outside the realm of being successful. In itself, the phrase *successful and usual* connotes dichotomy—the "either you are or are not" proposition of achievement. Disease prevention and health promotion are commonly framed in terms of preventing decline and optimizing function through behavioral change. An aim for a group or community may be set without portraying coincident individual achievement of a specific aim as success or the lack thereof as failure. Yet in aging, given its moral and religious antecedents, introducing the dichotomous notion of accomplishing success in avoiding the usual implies failure. Situating the meaning of being old in America in current yet historically aware context creates the possibility of failure. The connections that link understanding disease, particularly disease in which behavior is implicated, to moral matters of behavior and moral life perceive the presence of such disease or functional decline—the usual or expected ends of aging—as non-accomplishment at best and failure at worst.

What then are the implications of failing at being old? Failure, the usual state of being old, is logically related to the presence of disease. From that presence stems the experience of the disease as being ill, having symptoms through which the disease is apprehended, and requiring some form of curative or palliative treatment. Likely in that experience, being old and being ill are inextricably intermingled, each becoming part of the other state of being and eventually becoming indistinguishable. Even in our highly biomedically inclined society, dying of old age—as a disease would end a life in eventual organ damage and failure—is still offered as logical reasoning for death at very old chronological age. Only very old age by birth date replaces biomedically informed arguments of disease and cessation of function in the organs and cells. This causal argument for death stands apart from cellular senescence and understandings of the work of tissues and organs over an organism's biological life span. Rather, such an argument seems emblematic of the social conundrum of being old and ill placed in the historical circumstance of shifting knowledge and mores.

The meaning and images of being ill meld with capacity and function at any age. Incapacity relates back to experiential manifestations of disease—commonly held as symptoms rather than the signs that must be appraised by someone knowledgeable of disease—and to its impact in daily life. What one feels and what one can do in the face of minor acute illness or significant serious or chronic illness shapes perceived threat and imbalance. Further, externally perceived capacity and distress frames responses of others to the individual identified as ill. Response in care and concern reflects understanding of how capacity and distress are linked to personal impact of the disease and its treatment.

Introducing visual hallmarks of being old amplifies and complicates impressions of capacity and distress in illness. Our sense of what older adults can tolerate in disease and treatment contracts as our shared beliefs about the impact of the nexus of age and disease expands. That tension fosters a socially constructed understanding around being old and ill mediated by relationally perceived age and social meaning embedded in the disease. It matters how old and consequently how fragile you are and how socially threatening your illness is in constructing meaning implied by the state of being old and ill. For example, a person seen to be very old—at this writing, my gauging of that threshold is approximately older than eighty-five or ninety years—who has a disease understood to be ominous and opaque in its treatment—cancer and now Alzheimer's disease are among the most common, as they match the frequency of cardiovascular diseases—is more likely understood as despairing, suffering, and dying (Ferri et al. 2005; Patterson 1987). The tensions among age, disease, and tolerance issues impressionistic understanding arbitrated by proximity.

Out of these tensions emerges an existential time line balancing the tensions against an infirm ground of expectation, desire, and possibility (Kagan 1997). Decisions in health and health care are generally portrayed as the evaluation of cognitively bound information at a single point in time followed by an active judgment. In reality, I think few would describe decisions about health so calculatingly or discretely. Instead, a personal sense of health and decisions around health and adherent social care—more common with aging and introduction of chronic, age-associated disease—is far more emotional and fluid. Worry, fear, avoidance, vigor, joy, and other emotional sensations of embodiment intercede in that imagined cognition of decision making. Iterative embodied learning of desires, preferences, responses, and patterns shape that intercession as it winds through decades of life and daily living. Small distinctions—especially related to the prospect of illness and symptoms—are made in gauging the rightness of a decision or a set of choices made in health over the time of illness. For example, an older person who has experienced chronic illness may face a new diagnosis with that experience in mind. The new illness is compared with prior embodied knowledge and tracked as it evolves over time (Kagan 1997). External information about the disease and its presence as illness with varying bodily sensations is coupled with belief about self and illness in the expectations for and notions of a personal future. Thresholds for what can be tolerated or embraced are set and reset as the evocative background of daily life and an integrated sense of living evolve (Kagan 1997).

Daily living is ephemeral, establishing patterns and trends, shifting over time (Kagan 1997). Expectations, aims, and desires are altered as we age and accumulate experiences. The sensations and perceptions of a moment are tempered with a sense of the future and what it might hold. The influence of interplay between present and future appears easily in realms of attaining positive milestones such as college graduation, a new job, or retirement. The tension of present cost to future gain is clear and makes the decision to continue clear as well. Complexity of age-related dysfunction or illness often conjures fears of loss, dependence, burden, and dying. Fears of death in and of itself, though, recede as its capacity to pose relief grows against experience realized as unacceptable or intolerable. Such an equation evolves rapidly, often shifting remarkably over the course of hours or days. My patients commonly say to me, "It is a good day, but yesterday was awful," or "This afternoon is better than the morning was for me."[1] Simply stated estimations of the present tense evaluate the general quality of today for that person at this time in this context.

A narrative of daily living under thresholds and within future promise in very late chronological life vividly illustrates this present-tense evaluation. I came across the following story while searching for other related materials on the Internet. A California resident, Mr. Napolitano, at two different times recorded his story of being old and then having cancer in his local newspaper, *The Palisadian-Post*. A reporter visited Mr. Napolitano, whose first name is Joe, on the occasion of his 105th birthday: "I asked Joe how he felt, 'I feel good today,' he said, lighting up his pipe. 'I don't take any pills or medicine and I don't have any aches or pains, just old-age wear. I want to die like my grandfather back in Italy. He was ninety-seven and he smoked a pipe up until a week before he died. He wasn't sick or anything; he just didn't want to live anymore'" (Bruns 2004).

Later, after surgery for cancer, Mr. Napolitano wrote a letter to the editor: "I'm now feeling fine. I can still pass the DMV tests for driving. No glasses needed. Late last year, however, a tumor developed near my appendix and colon. It grew to the size of a tennis ball. The question was whether I should leave it to chance or undertake a dangerous operation. My general practice doctor, Roberta Smith, called in surgeon Dr. William Hutchinson, who lives here in the Palisades. He sent me to St. John's Hospital for several tests" (Napolitano 2005). After offering details of the surgery, Mr. Napolitano goes on to say, "Since the surgery my appetite has been great. I even tend to overeat sometimes. My favorite foods are lamb chops, fresh frozen vegetables and pastas of all shapes. I love pork but don't use it because it's loaded with water so that the flavor is gone. No beef, no chicken" (Napolitano 2005). In this statement, at once pragmatic and amusing in its confident preferences, Mr. Napolitano reframes the experience of cancer and portrays what he values in daily life and evaluates quality in his experience of it. He summarizes: "Now I'll put down my pipe and look over my Iliff neighborhood and friends. I've been surprised at how many friends I have with great appreciation" (Napolitano 2005).

The formula of the individual present in a specific moment in a specific context is transitory. With advancing age and experience, given the inexorability of a stable or progressive condition like cancer, that individual must gauge present experience and context in time and expectation. The future that seems temporarily secure and the experience tolerable may seem markedly different if expectations or experience change. Older adults' narratives of shifts in illness experienced over time reflect the gauging and evaluating that may lie behind a trend of days when— rather than "this afternoon is better than this morning"—the days are rated as exceeding thresholds and without relief or direction, as in "each day is no better than yesterday."

Mr. Cahn,[2] a man in his eighth decade of life who was a retired scientist and executive diagnosed with a sinus cancer, offered this narrative during a study of symptom experience:[3]

Well it's not been bad until the last year, where the sinus cancer has really progressed. And this thing is a hole in my face . . . and bandages . . . cosmetic . . . yeah covers all over my face. And . . . uh . . . the other things. Well it's gonna kill me. I know that. Uh . . . it's painful . . . it requires a lot of exotic treatments which may or may not work, which is why I'm here. Well because it is progressing at a fairly rapid rate. I had . . . well eight years ago . . . I had a maxillectomy [removal of part of the upper jaw, bone behind the cheek nearest the nose]. And it seemed cured and six years later it reappeared. Just [manage] day to day. I don't have much choice. Well, uh, eating for example. Is an ordeal. I don't like to eat with people. Because it [food] sorta slips out. So . . . I don't eat with people. Well I don't go out in public a lot. With this, uh, you know, bandage here. Well, my wife. She's important—married forty-two years. I'm a baseball fan. I watch a lot of baseball. Particular fan of the San Francisco Giants. I watch a lot of TV. Don't do much reading. I can't seem to concentrate.

Mr. Cahn vividly portrays his dilemma. Words made terse by the way his mouth is disfigured by sinus cancer illustrates aspects of daily life made intolerable by the effects of that cancer played out against his perennial sources of personal pleasure. His evaluation is tangible and temporal. He frames his story with time at the outset and ends with his own capacity. Mr. Cahn is easily imagined having a very different story a year or two prior to the description he offered me that day.

Mrs. Eck, Mr. Napolitano, and Mr. Cahn offer different stories of threshold and expectation that provide essential perspective on the tension of socially and culturally mediated impressions of being old and having cancer and the reality of individual experience that is today so common and familiar to many American families. We live our lives today in the context of an aging society. Changing demographics—and the rapid growth of older age groups—and the technological capacity for cancer treatment run sharply against socially embedded, shared, and embellished understandings of what it means to be old, and especially what it means to be old and have cancer. We more easily adapt to the stories of successful aging—the positive stereotypes of the octogenarian marathoner or the nonagenarian college graduate—that give us hope for late life unencumbered. We bridle against the notion that late life brings increased risk of disease and illness, disability, and altered function. Perhaps it is a primal response that speaks to innate survival mechanisms and aversion to thoughts of our own mortality, but stories that lack the pivotal point at which the war can be judged won and done seem less easily assimilated. Thus, while Mr. Napolitano's story garnered local newspaper coverage for the length and wisdom of his life as he lived it, Mr. Cahn and Mrs. Eck were eulogized in death, though their stories were no less triumphant or wise than his. Perspective on the tension comes then in understanding their stories in social context. There is nuance within each narrative, subtleties tied to preferences and lessons of lives mostly lived, and demands of the moment framed against a personal future. But social reaction and interest is predicated in previously constructed understandings of meaning that predate the way older people live today. Fundamentally, as one ages, a sense of one's own future accommodates a sense of personal mortality with the understanding that life is not a series of endless balances. The point on which that understanding balances moves with temporal features of illness, symptoms, and function. The lives of older people that are lived today, and not yesterday's understandings of what it means to be old, presage resolution of the tension between shared social understanding and emerging meaning of what it means to be old and have cancer. As that tension, and the shifts in demography, technology, and culture that generate it, abate, possibilities for aligning social understandings of what it means to be old and have cancer with the daily realities of those who live that life along with readily apparent revision needed in health and social care might become possible.

Chapter 3
Paradox
Cancer and Aging in America

Cancer and old age in America coalesce in an existential paradox. Human experience, the realities of aging, and proximate mortality play out against the reification of emerging science, investment in curative biomedicine, and the hopes of immortality. Our external objectification of personal health is supported by exalted belief in cellular and molecular biomedicine. Senescence, aging, and age-related disease are approached cognitively as if they collectively constitute a problem to be solved. Cancer has long been constituted as a cognitive puzzle, elevated to the level of national policy when Richard Nixon declared war on cancer (Sporn 1996). The virtue of the war is unassailable. To eradicate diseases that render so much suffering is fundamentally good. Nonetheless, the perspective of war leaves holes, events, and concerns unaddressed. This martial metaphor and an adherent cognitive puzzle of cancer for older adults can only be pieced together against the background of an aging society. Even if the war were won, in such an aging society, genetically predetermined mortality would win out in the last analysis. The war on cancer, as metaphor and as policy, generally neglects the inextricable link between advancing age and cancer. It then cannot approach the experience of cancer beyond the bounds of disease, leaving unexamined the realm of living with cancer that extends those boundaries.

We live lives that are no larger and no smaller than our surmounting tribulations of daily life, working toward dreams and goals, weathering crisis and tragedy, and celebrating milestones. In general, we age existentially as we do biologically, though often not in parallel. We pause to consider the nature and limits of existence and strive to develop science to help us understand increasingly detailed questions about the physical world. At the same time, we fully engage in aspects of daily life that are not scientific, outlining life narrative with enjoyment of humanistic, aesthetic facets of that existence. Being old and having cancer captures the manifold, often diametric tensions of more broadly drawn human existence in a developed society. This chapter outlines the enigmatic paradox emerging through social appropriation of scientific dominance in discourse on aging and the associated diseases as it is positioned against aging physically, psychologically, and socially; the existential nature of being old; and the experience of disease as part of life.

The news media, driven in part by a culture reifying the dominance of youth, influences public impressions of science as it addresses aging, creates the idea of "antiaging," and becomes the premier source of solution. The media report endless bits of science that impart an antiaging aura to many health reports. Popular interpretations of antiaging science abound. Recently, for example, the local NBC News crawl posted the caption "Apples may help prevent Alzheimer's" in a regurgitation of a two-month-old scientific paper on the value of quercetin, an antioxidant found in apples, and its effects on rat neurons.[1] The question of thin relevance for apples, quercetin, human neurons, and Alzheimer's disease, while addressed in the story, is almost incidental. I investigated that relevance in other presentations of the same story. Every online write-up and newsy sound bite I reviewed implies that apples, particularly red apples, which contain more quercetin, would be a useful addition to any person's diet. In that slice of antiaging science speak, apples seem destined to become a dietary mainstay. The express argument, of the sort so common today in indiscriminate dissemination of partial scientific information, claimed that ingestion of red apples could not hurt and might help. It simultaneously delimited specific application with the implication that these apples might help *fight* cancer if eaten daily. Many news reports even offered the kind suggestion of other foods rich in quercetin (e.g., cranberries, blueberries, and onions among others) if you don't like apples. Though there are likely no disadvantages to eating more apples, the promise of protection from a fearsome disease and the inferred obviation of aging suggest thwarting the battle before it reaches fever pitch. The claims, of course, are dilute at best. Yet that weak retort to aging and associated disease is in fact what made the item newsworthy.

The struggle between the inevitability of aging and the science that hopes to mitigate it is made real in the story's newsworthiness and fantastical in contrast to daily life. We can, through lived experience, apprehend that apples alone will not ward off cancer, Alzheimer's disease, or any other condition. The avuncular adage "An apple a day keeps the doctor away,"[2] variously attributed to a nursery rhyme or Benjamin Franklin, can be an abstract motto of a simple health-giving diet or a literal maxim of dietary apple intake. The desire to infer scientific and specific propositions that relate precise dietary intake to disease prevention and antiaging abounds. The wish itself, though, is discordantly abstract. The experience of living our individual lives remains more complex and less controlled than the simple articulation of one's desire to prevent disease and avoid aging. Family history, presenting genotypes not as yet amenable to pinpoint modification, and life lived, before knowledge of prevention for specific disease could be applied in behaviors such as eating apples, cast large and unwieldy shadows on that desire.

In the months preceding this writing, I spoke at the University of Pennsylvania Institute on Aging twenty-fifth anniversary annual retreat opposite Vincent Cristofalo, a bellwether bench scientist in aging and gerontology whose immense stature in the scientific community at the University of Pennsylvania and beyond is almost incomprehensible. I gave a talk titled "The Scientific Import of Embedded Social Constructions of Being Old and Having Cancer," only slyly subtitled "How Bench Scientists Can Help Reconstruct Outmoded Social Icons of Aging." Dr. Cristofalo spoke lucidly on directions for science in longevity and senescence. I recall thinking that his approach to interpreting bench science in aging for an interdisciplinary audience of widely varying familiarity with that discipline was remarkably adept and understated. He avoided broad claims about senescence and the human condition and instead built a careful argument that taught as much as it proposed. Though we both spoke on current and salient issues in aging, I was struck by a gulf between the knowledge and the understanding of cells that Dr. Cristofalo compellingly represented and twined into emerging science, and the socially shared and communicated notions of aging and being old that I carved out. Aging cells and aging individuals seemed for a long time to be alien entities, confronting each other in a paradoxical world where science is increasingly seen as subcellular investigation and where inquiry into human behavior and society is often termed "soft science." I came away from that retreat sharply aware that forward progress compelled work toward resolving this paradox. Knowledge requires ever widening frames that compose relevance, utility, and direction.

The paradox of science and social experience played out more specifically in my readings some months later. The experience of speaking at the Institute on Aging retreat was followed by reading well-regarded journalist Stephen Hall's *Merchants of Immortality* (Hall 2003), whose lurid cover is obviously inspired by the graphics of science fiction films of the 1950s, and inscribed to me by a colleague who had offered it as a gift symbolic of our shared interest in aging. My colleague's inscription to me reads, "To the eternal human quest for the 'fountain of youth'—our ultimate calling in health care." The idea of a fountain of youth attracted and puzzled me in my often somewhat naïve reverence for what can be learned and comprehended in contemplating and studying advancing age. But Hall's book, with its eye-catching cover and my colleague's perplexing inscription, sat unread for many months on my bedside table. Would it tell me more of youth and less of age than I imagined, or would it challenge my humanistic valuation of advancing age as a pure good in and of itself?

Eventually, I read it. The contrast of the book's content, my colleague's inscription, and Hall's remarkably personal epilogue preoccupied me. The story woven by Hall about the particular scientific pursuit of immortality began with the Hayflick limit[3] and extended to science and consequent debates about cloning (Hall 2003). The fountain of youth appeared as almost absurdly folkloric pitched before a story that, while it told of legendary scientific discovery, was innately and importunately human. As he told of the discovery, Hall—perhaps because he is a journalist appealing to a popular audience—uncovered the fierce competition, political backbiting, and brutish territoriality that often is said to play alongside emergence of new knowledge.

In the end, the fountain of youth did not seem terribly improbable paired with the image of immortality that Hall conveyed in his book (2003). They both felt as relatively unattainable as the author more compellingly portrayed the story of cellular senescence, which began to appear to me, as I recalled past conversations with bench scientists, more like exploration of the moon than the discovery of the fountain of youth. The moon is an everyday presence with everyday effects: the lunar cycle, moonlight, and physical properties of mass, space, and orbit. As we develop better and better tools to explore it, more information is known about it and at a more detailed level. In fact, knowledge gained from specialized studies emerging from exploration of the moon—inquiry into weightlessness and health, for example—offer direct application to human life. But the moon itself does not change. Aging seems, in all likelihood, to be akin to the moon. Its features are primarily predetermined. Modification of those features implies only that—modification, not reversal or removal. As our tools improve and our knowledge expands, science derived from the study of senescence will apply to facets of human life, but aging will remain.

Immortality is a fantasy of the fountain of youth that likely becomes less appealing as one ages. While there are many people who prove the exception with their fascination with or fixation on regaining lost youth, most adults progress in intrinsic knowing of self, realizing that a return to youth is impossible and indeed undesirable. Youth, in all of its advantages and disadvantages, is lost in maturation, although some enjoyable and coveted characteristics of youth such as physical prowess may be grieved. I am constantly fascinated by individual reactions to the desire for an exceptionally long life—almost certainly to be in excess of 100 years now in developed nations. I commonly offer in everyday conversation with many different people my hope that I will live to the age of 120 years. Alternately, I ask people I meet casually how long they would like to live. Responses I receive to these prompts are strikingly dissimilar to the ethos of antiaging and show little infatuation with any but minor aspects of youthful vigor.

Individuals very deliberately contemplate what advanced chronological age would mean in their everyday lives. Rather than connoting a life couched in images of the fountain of youth, reactions are predicated on far more nuanced and personal substrates. Many people who respond declare very old age undesirable. Some speak of it with imagined connotations of frailty and loss, and some often speak of disease common in their family histories. These responses are less common than I had imagined; painful stories of loved ones in the ninth or tenth decades of their lives sentenced to suffering and lingering death by disease, iatrogenesis, and poverty are rare. Likewise, biblical denotation and express belief in divine directives are uncommon. Absent desire for extensive longevity seems far more personal in much of American life.

Distaste for exceptionally long life is more often sharpened by thoughts of outliving one's cohort or by a fundamental fatigue and disinterest in the world. It is as though individuals will approach life as a finite entity when not pressed by immediate fears of illness or death. Not *too* long a life is the prevailing sentiment. The qualifying use of *too* is emphasized. What is too long? Too long seems far more connected to relationships, interest, and energy than to disease and science. Disease, illness, and lost capacity and function are certainly embedded in what constitutes too long. The line that extends from disease to dysfunction at some point intersects with interpersonal relations, interest in life, and embodied energy. Individuals understand intrinsic thresholds and gauge experience of health and illness against those thresholds to judge—consciously or not—what is not tolerable as thresholds of embodiment are exceeded. But it is only in intersection with what is valued in daily life that the personal definition of a distant mortality rises up and becomes relevant. Immortality and aging collide as fantastical thoughts meet daily reality. Antiaging is relegated to the growing domain of physical image, cosmetic preparations, and superficial aesthetic adjustment. Physical fitness is ironically less present than one might expect. Nonetheless, immortality alone appears disagreeable. Perhaps this is because daily life is inherently narrative, encompassing the passing of time and a sense of order that must end whether at the end of the day, the year, or the lifetime. Despite reviling old age in at least paradigmatic visual impressions and infatuation with delaying visual hallmarks of old age, perhaps human understanding of aging is oddly built upon the hidden inevitability of death, or the inarguable promise of it at the very least.

The paradoxical tension between fantasies of antiaging and a semblance of immortality and the aging life course with its developmental milestones may be contextually derived—a product of a culture laden with Protestant ethics and commingled cultural precepts—or an innate aversion to a sense of meaning and relationship that seems perpetually human. Perhaps it is both, twined together, creating a range of expressions across communities, with some individuals at one extreme or the other and most spread across narrative time and personally imagined life spaces. The constrained response to an imagined extraordinarily long life may be created in the temporal knowledge that threats of loss, dysfunction, and death are publicly associated with very old age. And perhaps the response would change if those sorts of threats were mitigated. Alternatively, perhaps the response of not desiring an excessively long life is innate. Is it possible that the envisaged end of one's life must be somewhat abstract to be comprehensible? The relevance of life and the meaning of one's life might necessitate clearly drawing the point where aims are judged achieved or unachievable and accomplishment outweighs enthusiasm.

Although the ideal of living a long life is cherished in many ways beyond science that encompass religion and folklore, the obverse idea of having lived too long gauged against a particular life and contemporary context is equally relevant. Think of Washington Irving's story of Rip Van Winkle with its sad entailment of being out of time and place.[4] The children's novel *Tuck Everlasting* (Babbitt 1985), which was later made into a film, addresses life achievement and accomplishment. It juxtaposes achievement against the adolescent wish for immortality, with the fictional convenience of an immortal family. In the film, the heroine is offered immortality and love and declines them in favor of a mortal life. The film ends as the narrator says, "You don't have to live forever, you just have to live" (Lieber 2002). The enduring nature of folklore and literature underscores the paradoxical relationship between science and belief and between aging and understanding. So the dissonance between immortality, contained in contemporary scientific housing, and aging, in a human life course, divides the factual—typified by science—and the ineffable—revealed in humanism.

Returning to Hall's *Merchants of Immortality* (2003), I find what I think is his understanding of the dissonance of immortality and aging together with embedded issues of being old in the epilogue. Hall's book begins with the Hayflick limit and ends with cloning and stem cells. It is all impersonal and scientific. However, his story called "Finitude" in the epilogue is very personal. Hall writes about his old, ill mother and the care she receives. In describing his mother's predicament and his reaction to it, Hall dwells for a moment in the very human experience of finding meaning in loss before going on to reflect again on the industry of immortality—regenerative medicine and life extension technology—and the current sociopolitical environment and its appointed guardians of the ethics of that industry. But it is Hall's moment of looking profoundly at his mother and her work of being old and ill and striving to recover that captured my interest. Regardless of how much evidence science accretes, can it succeed in altering the "moon" of human aging by changing aspects of its cellular mechanisms? Or will there always be that finitude to which Hall alluded (2003)?

Being old and having cancer highlights this question and funnels paradox into a personally apprehended, potentially threatening mirage that is neither as horrific as popular conception nor as easy as some individual experience. The dissonance among our imaginings, rapidly evolving scientific understandings, and realities of being old and having cancer strikes at our inability to reconcile issues of mortality, dependence, and function. Youth and imagined youthful dimensions of function are a metric against which we measure and then perhaps value old age. What is old is defined as opposite to or dichotomous with youth. Visual and text media surround us with messages about material aspects of youth that may then be transmogrified into what is old. This connection is distanced and abstracted in images of consumable goods and their supposed impact on the consumer. The connection is clearly important as consumption and the consumer tell us a great deal about constructions of social value and economic import. But exclusive focus on what automobile says young as opposed to old, for example, offers relatively evanescent understanding and avoids distasteful prospects of imagined states of being old and ill. The cascade to mortality through altered function and dependence is more substantive, where inquiry reveals more fundamental notions of being and meaning in old age and illness.

The overt metric of youth confines and stagnates discourse around old age as youth is made normative and old age becomes the exception. Visually apt and material references to material possession adapt easily to this metric. Youthful self is bought and sold at a superficial level as it is mediated by intricate generational ideals, social pressures, and economic values. Old self is a harder sell. A recent news story on Buick automobiles and their contradictory image of youth and wealth underscores that nothing automotive says middle class and old like Buick in America (Petersen 2005). The story uncovers that the hard sell is in the converse case—to which the story only alludes—that Buick is struggling to sell in America with that image (Petersen 2005). While this case is sharply drawn through cross-cultural contrast and the iconic status of automobiles across generations, it nonetheless illustrates the relative invisibility of being old. A rather light news story embosses messages of advertising on viewers' memories, conjuring nostalgia through replayed Buick advertisements of decades past and creating cross-national questions as China is shown glorifying a discarded American material image. Old, as the exception in a normative social discourse focused on youth, is then a source of tension in this and other illustrations—whenever and wherever they surface. Thinking about and attending to issues of aging and being old then requires greater concentration and movement away from the normative and toward the alternative.

The conflict between what is socially normative—youth—and what is demographically common—old—places at odds social discourse, individual and familial experience, and economic forces. Ironically, maintaining social construction of old as exceptional and specialized is demographically incorrect and pragmatically constrictive. The anticipated aging of the baby boom generation by chronological definitions of fifty-five, sixty, or sixty-five years of age instigates excursive musings on the power of their coming to old age. While their number compels attention, current focus on them as a generally highly functional and independent generation avoids the emotionally charged strength of their parents' generations, which are approximately identified as being comprised of those born before 1931. They are those who lived through World War II as adults, adolescents, and school-age children and are commonly and quite sardonically referred to as the "matures" or the "mature generation." This wry appellation suggests so much about an American approach to being old. That they would be called mature, while their legacy generation carries the word *baby* as a generational label, connotes unerring emphasis on youth and a generational divide. That divide leaves the so-called mature generation in a place of further exclusion and fruitless quest for solutions typifying another dimension of paradox in aging.

Those of the mature generation, the generation that predates and recalls World War II in great detail, are now classified as middle- or old-old by gerontologists as they have exceed ages of seventy-five and eighty years (Schuman and Rodgers 2004; Munnell 2004). Many of them constitute the most rapidly growing demographic age group in our society—the old-old—as they live past eighty-five years of age and in many cases approach the centenary mark (Scommegna 2004; Himes 2003). Many of this generation defy stereotypes of longevity and function as they surpass the current life expectancy of eighty years, still living independent lives and engaging in a variety of activities (Himes 2003; Scommegna 2004). But with very late life comes an increased risk of multiple and chronic changes in health status and necessary instrumental and social support. The needs of these more fragile members of the generation and the pressures their needs visit on an unprepared society vastly outweigh expository musings on baby boom aging and the change that generation is promised to wreak in our society (Lee and Skinner 1999; Munnell 2004). Current demands for structures and systems to address prospective and immediate health and social need are felt acutely by many families caring for the most fragile of this group and by communities overburdened by growing numbers of the old-old. Being old and having an illness like cancer, especially when it coexists with other chronic health and functional limitations, creates profound and lasting need over time. This extension of demography and illness reflects possible and even probable extremity in unmet health and social needs.

Study and practice in aging and illness have consistently upheld and currently maintain the notion of aging as not normative but the exception. To a great extent, I think the modern American allopathic approach to care that employs specialization and often subspecialization emphasizes this perspective. Health and social care for older adults is broadly defined as generalist guided care, using services of specialists in gerontology and geriatrics as needed to resolve or—less commonly—prevent problems. The immediate socioeconomic pressures of systems designed to deliver health and social care not withstanding, study and practice in aging upholds the larger social constructions that place old age and the process of aging—as opposed to popularized notions of antiaging—in the background. The exception has its advantage in connotations of that which is special and apart. The advantage extends until it runs the limit of current demographics, often localized as immediate communal pressures on systems and infrastructure. The dichotomy of youth and old age is far less advantageous to the latter, as old age is almost necessarily placed in subordinate opposition, thereby losing any cachet of being separate and apart, with the overriding image of cumulative loss and being less-than.

The central challenge then is to recast being old and having cancer in the cycle of the life span without exclusion to late life. Titian's painting *The Three Ages of Man*[5] impels me to define this challenge. In a space that is both timeless and culturally transcendent, Titian's old man sits in the background of the painting gently and poignantly fondling two skulls. The European antecedents of dominant American cultural understandings of aging are unmistakable. The dominance of masculinity and a Protestant European ethos supports the manifestation of physical fragility, sadness, and impending death in the picture of late life as much as it makes the feminine and other religious and cultural tradition invisible. The dominance Titian captured as his backgrounded old age and foregrounded youth echoes in contemporary directions for study and practice in aging. Shaping trends in inquiry and care from the most subcellular approaches through large-scale populational and communal programs require delineation of moral blind spots issued in the emblematic paradox of youth and old age, science, and the experience representative of being old and having cancer in America.

Most fundamentally, the schism between diagnosis and death, stated by biomedical science as incidence and mortality, represents the human scale of the paradox. Diagnosis is of disease and increasingly of cells and their components. The disease that is diagnosed is clearly attended by human experience, but its treatment is ever more focused on cellular and subcellular mechanisms. Death remains an inherently existential organismal event, enigmatic or mysterious depending on individual spiritual or other explanatory frames. We have invested endless resources and built vast structures to make science the solution in aging, couched as a problem, and cancer, defined as disease. Investment in science creates strength as knowledge builds, collective and crosscutting characteristics emerge, and explanations coalesce. In the emerging and increasingly obverse case, reliance on science leaves lingering desire for what is human and individual. We struggle with scientific paradigms that underscore knowing what is of the group, what is collective, and what is different between groups. The most immediate example of this is clinical trials to test the effects of medications. The most basic aim of such trials is to give nearly identical groups a drug and a placebo and measure the difference in the disease under study. As a society, we place faith in this science of the collective—threatened now by a series of adverse events and consequent litigation cast in the realm of health care errors and safety. Still, as recipients of care that is driven by such science, we want to be known and treated as individuals. The war on cancer, as it was declared by Nixon, epitomizes such investment in science of the collective (Sporn 1996). Cancer, understood as a disease of cells, recognizes that human cells are fundamentally alike from human to human. Our current cellular and subcellular grasp on cancer is arguably unparalleled. Winning the war on cancer—as a disease but perhaps not as an illness—seems so much more possible than before the genomic era. In this war, surviving as an organism, which was threatened by the disease, is the only possible plan of action. The plan is as real for individuals as it is for society. Winning the war then mandates that the disease is conquered for the individual as it is for society. The scientific armamentarium triumphs over cells that behave in destructive and lethal ways. Surviving is defined in biomedical terms of years of life after diagnosis. Succumbing to the disease connotes failure. Language of failure pervades cancer care, for example, where the person is said to fail treatment. The treatment driven by collective science does not fail the individual. This perspective is not, however, monolithic. For example, recent emphasis on research and care for survivors—defined as anyone who has been diagnosed with cancer—reassures with reaffirmed rather than trailing emphasis on the person and within-group variation. And yet, as old age connotes a more proximate personal mortality and the psychic existential coming to terms with that mortality, the war on cancer fundamentally and inexorably excludes those who are old and face death, whether from cancer or—more likely—not, regardless of battles won.

The space between incidence and mortality is living—the drudgery and joy of daily living that is more often influenced than defined by cancer as it is experienced in an array of chronic conditions such as arthritis and illnesses such as heart disease and dementia. Those who are young and do not innately perceive a proximate personal mortality live a daily life in which cancer is overriding—their purview is to engage in battle with the aim and the hope that winning the battles will end the war. Older individuals who recognize proximate but not immediate mortality face more intricate, nuanced choices limited by life stories in which time is limited. Treatment for cancer must fit into a life mostly lived in which daily living may include myriad values, interests, and activities as well as competing health and social needs. What is waged as war on a young individual's cancer becomes a fine balancing act that must account for individual experience and meaning found in the life of the person who has the cancer, and for an older person facing cancer in a life mostly lived, curing or controlling the cancer itself.

Chapter 4
Scientific Import and Influence

Social understandings of being old and having a disease like cancer, embedded in our collective consciousness, seem at first to have little direct influence on basic and clinical sciences. The intellectual distance between a common or shared image, such as that of pain, suffering, and social isolation often conjured by the phrase "an old man with cancer," and cellular and molecular science aimed at determining specific elements of carcinogenesis appears wide. Social science documents how we understand and what we construct to be common elements of collective human experience. That offers a vantage point from which cells and molecules are literally and figuratively unseen. Conversely, cellular and molecular science exists in a plane where human experience and social phenomena are unseen. That which is apparently invisible attracts attention; it becomes most intriguing and consequential to explore.

This chapter aims to dissect the import of understandings, socially shared, of being old and having cancer for the basic and clinical sciences, carried out at cellular, subcellular, and molecular levels, to understand the origins of cancer as a disease of old cells, and to better its treatment. The dissection is undertaken with the assumption that the social context in which science is designed and conducted must be articulated as a metric for judging the import of adjacent social phenomena. The central analysis is posited after the paradigmatic issues inherent in this exploration are discussed and the nature of social phenomena and the implied elements of social construction used here are detailed. The aging demographics of our society set up the exploration of images in social construction of what it means to be old and what it means to be old and ill in our society, with emphasis on the physical body. Implications of that construction in issues and consequences of ageism in science with reference to being old and having cancer follow. The nexus of exploring that experience in clinically promising science is played out against a vast backdrop. Perceptions of need, images of mortality, and desires for longevity impinge upon projected future constructions that may or may not fit a scientific continuum.

Science is a human enterprise and as such exists within the society in which the science itself is conducted. Inherently then, science is also a social phenomenon in and of itself and can only be fully understood in its aims, design, methods, and analysis through exploration of its social context. Social context lends credence to particular lines of inquiry, weight to specific methodological streams, and value to findings that fall within the frame of desired format and substance, following what has been viewed as credible and noteworthy. What is valued is conversely framed in terms of value for some good. That good must be delineated in a manner that makes clear that the pursuit of knowledge that supports that good is indeed good itself, then, and worthy of effort and resources. To a great extent, what determines the value and worth of a specific science and the actual conduct of that science becomes a Möbius strip of inextricably intertwined and interlocking reasoning. For example, as the reciprocal technologies and methods that enable understanding of the human genome have expanded and advanced, the science of human genomics for basic and translational purposes have become increasingly valued. Though this value is not without internal debate (e.g., around cloning technologies as an application of human genomics), the promise and pride of this general realm of science grows in power and repute. Rhetoric now extends from genomic science to consideration of genomic cures, as it were, to diseases that plague humankind and even aging itself.

The value given science shapes the conduct of science. As science requires resources and human effort to be completed, the act of conducting science demands appropriation of the resources deemed necessary to complete the act. Science demands a laboratory or field for inquiry, tools for collecting and analyzing data, and people to carry out the activities of design, data collection, analysis, and dissemination. Appropriation of the necessary resources, as any resources are finite in nature, must be made through decisions about which science is deserving of them. Sciences viewed as valuable to society are more likely to be supported with resources and therefore more likely to be undertaken.

As science is a human enterprise, scientists generally face political realities as part of the social context in which they operate and which then shapes science. In America, that reality is most evident in federal funding priorities for science and in criteria for judging scientific work. The political elements of social context tend toward conservation of the familiar and replicable. While creativity is admirable, overabundance of it without clear and close antecedents, and a continuity with that earlier work, is likely perceived to lessen scientific import, increase political risk, and jeopardize success in funding and peer review. This political nature in science is, to a certain extent, imparted by the view of science as a collective, authorless body of knowledge.

Science is viewed as an evolutional body of knowledge ordered in what is known and how it is known. Progress in science can generally be seen retrospectively, across a period of time in which incremental change in knowledge is easily apprehended. The appraisal of progress depends on the complexity of the science, the level at which it is in fact appraised, and the expertise of the appraiser. Conversely, science is broadly understood in a particular moment from an explicit general perspective. That general perspective on which there is agreement within an area of science is the received view of that science. As science is a human undertaking, it is a subject of social context, consideration, and agreement. The received views of specific realms of science are products of that social process. The received view enables continued work within an area of science to continue through validation of direction and growth deemed valuable. That continued work, however, is generally undertaken in close proximity to science situated within the bounds of the received view.

Received views of science can become problematic when seemingly significant matters that involve science fall outside the bounds of those received views. Balance between creativity and continuity is implied by virtue of the received view and codified by political elements of social context. But is there a place in which societal change outstrips contemporary science and scientific thought to such an extent that balance in creativity and continuity cannot immediately be achieved? Creativity is necessary to advance scientific knowledge while continuity is indispensable to a body of knowledge that may be apprehended as logical and systematic. Nevertheless, the extremity of mismatched need and inquiry might only be resolved in a creative leap that appears discontinuous with current science. A creative leap to transcend the dissonant gap between knowledge and application in an area of human science may stretch the bounds of the received view and threaten political and peer credibility. Resolution of dissonance and lessening tension in credibility then seem at odds. Attenuating strain is perhaps most intriguing in the context of human science where consequences are personally sensible.

Human phenomena, when viewed within social science and then as inherently involving interaction, are remarkably complex. They are rather difficult to parse into broad areas of inquiry. While specifically defined questions that beget precisely shaped inquiry are easily apprehended, the realms into which they fit are less easily grasped. That grasp is dependent to a certain extent on paradigmatic assumptions about stance in science. Ontological questions of objective truth, experiential knowledge, and subjective reality all play out differentially in accordance with the substance implied by the scientific prism of the paradigm in which they are studied. Threading these different questions together, however, are common aspects of human interaction that center ontology of the phenomena and enable organization of episte-mological questions.

Human interaction can, in a fundamental sociological sense, be or-dered in relation to self, other, and context (Mead 1967). All interac-tions have "self" and "other" situated in a context. The distinction of self and other are imparted by the perspective of focus and experience. That perspective stems from the self while the one appraised is the other. Anything relevant to the interaction itself is context, whether tangible or intangible. Representations and abstractions of self, other, and context can then be ordered to describe a specific or general interaction and its attributes. An ordinary interaction, for example, one in which a person greets a new acquaintance, is bound in context of environment, society, power, relationship, and many other dimensions. While each greeting has particularly unique details, most can be abstracted into categories of self, other, and context that allow its description within that category of interaction. That description may then echo more persistent meanings attached to human interactions, meanings that background shared un-derstanding within the interaction itself.

Persistent meanings, shared among members of a group, assemble in social constructions of what that meaning is and how it influences the interaction. Those group members share meanings attached to being and place in social interaction. The meaning is ascribed though attri-butes or characteristics that are viewed in light of the varying importance imputed to them. Meaning is often readily perceived by calling to mind general human attributes such as gender or age that may be understood both as an element of self that is experienced and as a characteristic of others. Those ordinary attributes of being human also permit delinea-tion of a sense of an inner dimension and a shared or social dimension in the life world of a particular person. While the inner dimension of that person's life world is clearly interesting and of great consequence in health and illness, the discussion here focuses on the social dimension to illuminate themes and gaps in knowledge of what it is to be old and have cancer in our society.

Consequences of demographics and health are, in relation to advanc-ing age, usually outlined on a large scale of populations, communities, care entailed, and costs attached. Much is made of the demographics of our rapidly aging society, and inferences drawn from them, about neces-sarily large-scale challenges to health care and health care service deliv-ery (Cutler and Meara 1997; Hazzard 1997). In some manner, our aging population has become an icon in itself. Statistics that lay out astounding growth in the old-old population, explicate overwhelming increases in health care costs for older adults when compared with younger adults, and similarly overpowering facts are compelling (Cutler and Meara

1997). They transfix us—young or old, professional or lay person—in that they force our contemplation and challenge us to understand consequence on a human scale.

Being old in our society is to exceed the superficial myth that you are old at a preset chronological age, a birth date that fits some expectation of what one does in old age. Presently, we seem to be stuck on the cusp of a long-held national notion that there is a specific age at which one is old—perhaps retirement at sixty or sixty-five or being on Medicare at sixty-five. But that myth is buffeted by competing newer images of active adults over the age of sixty-five and catchphrases in the media like "Fifty is the new thirty." Meaning implied by those long-held and emerging images are the fabric of our socially constructed connotations of what it means to be old in our society—the feelings, ideas, and speculative ramifications conjured by this phrase. These understandings are myriad, ranging from positive images of cherished older friends and relatives to negative stereotypes and personal fears of dependence, isolation, and mortality.

So what lies at the core of the meaning of being old in relation to health, illness, and care specifically? For many in our society, including older adults and their professional and lay caregivers, core components might center on risk of or actual functional loss that exceeds some imagined boundary between social and personal independence and dependence. Independence and dependence must correlate to age in a socially appropriately manner.[1] Considering notions of independence across the life span, from infancy through adolescence and adulthood to late life, immediately captures that sense of the appropriate in simple care of ourselves (e.g., toilet use) and complex social behaviors (e.g., acquiring an education or applying the skills of an occupation). The network of lost function and ensuing need for care appears to hold special significance in late life without precise reference to what caused function to decline. The significance may rest in expectation, experience, or a socially mediated cycle drawing on many influences. Nevertheless care needs, in all of their practical and symbolic aspects, necessarily imply demand for care and the extent to which that demand is met. While families generally meet the bulk of need that is acknowledged, nurses commonly supply care that is technical or complex. Nurses also provide education that enables family caregivers to take on new levels or types of activities in their care of the older adult.

Nurses, in fact, are members of the single profession whose social contract, education, and skills span a continuum of need in late life. A focus on human responses to shifts from health to illness and back through recovery to new states of health intrinsically mandates an intimate sensibility of human experiences from the mundane, essential, and private to the emotional, cherished, and public. In late life, as function may fall away in disease and disuse, compensation for varying levels of function and restoration of what might be brought back becomes increasingly prominent. Nursing focuses in late life on function, from promoting healthy behaviors and suggesting practical adaptations to minimal decrement in function though supportive care that compensates for loss of basic, intimate functions such as bowel control and toileting. As risk for and actual functional losses expand, nursing actions intensify, becoming more intimate and human in a most fundamental sense. Eventually then, needs to be met through nursing care—whether directly or indirectly, as through family education—predominate in the array of care provided for the oldest old. Societal understandings of that care are shaped by meanings of what it is to be old, ill, and dependent on others for basic care.

The discomfort called up by meanings of being old, ill, and in need of care reflects back to what is fundamentally human in daily function. To be human is to move through space and time, functioning in a manner that desired actions are taken with effort that is largely unnoticed. Taken-for-granted function requires no effort because effort exerted is invisible. As increasing effort is required to compensate for lost function, invisibility is worn away. Functions basic to being human—speaking, eating, washing one's body, and toileting—surface as effort becomes visible. The obverse of the wearing away is the inverse invisibility of the care provided to compensate for the innate loss and of the person, family, or nurse providing that care. As care needs grow and become increasingly intimate, the care and those who provide it are caught in the discomfort the need connotes and become as invisible as the function itself was perceived to be.

Grasping the state of being old is an iterative, temporal discourse. It is evocative and, at the same time, ephemeral. While chronological age is always offered up as a marker of entering late life, the state of being old is less easily determined. Many disciplines approach the nature of being old from their varied, individual standpoints. Aging identity is popularly as well as scientifically explored in the changing body from senescent cells to antiaging remedies that address visible and socially disagreeable markers of advanced age. But do these explorations resonate with individual experience of aging and being old? Social and behavioral scientists and clinicians commonly examine evolving relationships. Changes in familial relationships, vocational or occupational role shifts, and other socially defined and perceived alterations in patterned interactions are frequently offered in conversations about topics considered relevant to aging and being old. Retirement from a job or professional position, emphasis on an avocation or hobby, establishing familial roles of grandparent or great-grandparent and widowhood are all notable topics in classic social gerontology.

As our society becomes more diverse in culture, economy, and life ways and simultaneously grows more aged, classically defined representations of being old—for instance, retirement from work outside the home—fit less well. They are superficial markers of shifting social constructions and hence feel incongruous or not completely in keeping with current experiences of being old. Previously commonplace and now increasingly unfavorable connotations captured by words such as *disengagement, detachment,* or *inutility* may not match impressions of active lives at levels from the intellectual and emotional to the highly physical, lived well into the eighth or ninth decade of life. Locating a less easily influenced element of meaning in being old is then consequential. What exists beneath historically bound, impermanent, socially determined roles and positions and beyond issues of social identity?

Temporal expectation of mortality is an element of human psychosocial development that transcends specific theory and discerns the evolution in outlook with advancing age. As individuals age, they move from no awareness of mortality in early life through a sense of immortality in adolescence to a growing knowingness of personal and proximate mortality. This understanding of personal mortality that comes nearer with advancing age is uniquely human and normatively different from other points in life. The expectation of our own mortality is then necessarily temporal but not chronological in that it is not switched on at a specified age. That temporality then allows shifts in context and possibility. Familial longevity, advances in health care and biomedical science, and personal desire are all shaped by incremental historical, social, cultural, and personal forces. The temporal expectation of mortality, however, remains a constant point from which meaning is constructed.

Adding cancer to the experience of being old creates complexity in many ways and at many levels of meaning. Here historical implications of cultural elements such as religion are intertwined with current constructions of health, aging, and death. Prevailing social constructions of what it means to be old in our society entail shared understandings of health and aging, framed by a sense of mortality and the meaning of death. Similarly, what is denoted by temporal expectation of proximate mortality links to social constructions of what it means to have cancer. Cancer at any age is held to imply threat of death, with incident implication of anticipated death, pain, discomfort, and suffering. The connotations of having cancer are parallel to the meaning attached to being old in its less favorable social construction. The two states combined currently hold an additively unfavorable connotation.

Historical themes in being old and having cancer emerge as influential in shaping contemporary meaning and simultaneously serving as a contrasting counterpoint against which current experience is reflected. Our social history bears the marks of cultural and particularly Protestant religious thought on matters of aging, morality, and illness (Cole 1992). Accretion and evolution of notions of aging and its relation to morality and immorality layer meaning seen in contemporary notions of living well or poorly. Moral overtones color understandings of disease and illness, easily apprehended in common questions about what an individual did to contract or develop a disease. Those who live morally enjoy health and successful aging, then tragically but not unacceptably succumb to illness, generally absent particular social import, and proceed to a dignified death at a suitably advanced age. Images of successful aging (Rowe and Kahn 1987), despite being given scientific overtones as a physical and physiological process in gerontology literature, still carry moral shading. Conversely, immoral living begets disease and illness prototypically seen in images of decrepit old age. Many popular representations of old age are imbued with impressions of suffering dissipation induced by immoral thoughts and actions.

Being old and having cancer closely follows this sociocultural paradigm of moral influence on disease in late life (Leichter 2003). Implications of having lived long enough to accrue moral credit or lack thereof are threaded through images of having cancer as an adult. While immorality and cancer have historically held religious parallels, more modern-day images implicate specific behaviors. This part of the construction is quickly apprehended in stereotypes of lifelong smokers and in the popular affront to someone newly diagnosed with cancer, "So what did you do to get it?" The more time spent in an ill-chosen behavior, the greater the threat to immorality and the larger the decrement to the life span. The social stigmata of cancer are simply and profoundly compounded by being old.

Socially defined dichotomies are ordinarily constructed to make sense of seemingly simple but implicitly convoluted intellectual structures such as the process of aging and the human body. Aging, while it is a biologically continuous process, is practically dichotomized into young and old. A usual question describing an individual is, "Is she young or old?" A middle age is added only to create a normative point of reference that is neither too young nor too old in the appraiser's discernment. Middle age usually implies escaping the disadvantage of being too young or too old within certain situations. Even more classically, age is further dissected for discrete evaluation. The mind is dichotomized in relation to the body through Cartesian dualism; despite ballooning science that reveals intricate interrelationships, social images of human function and behavior persists in returning to the dualism. Thus the mind may be judged older or younger than the body in which it resides.

Deleterious effects of age and disease are then often associated with one aspect of the dichotomy or the other. Specifically in aging, this dualism creates compartments in which age and aging shape stereotypical images of late life. Combined, the young-old dichotomy and Cartesian dualism give simple shape and easily apprehended maxims to our understandings of aging and the body. Crossing from young to old creates specific vulnerabilities in the mind and the body. Social images of Alzheimer's disease, for example, easily illustrate what is habitually seen as an image of the old mind in a body either young or old in these intersected dichotomies.

Science aimed at revealing cellular and subcellular components of human phenomena that result in observable responses and behavior stands opposite dichotomies and value-laden images and stereotypes. Increasingly, science underscores that incremental change in biological human systems creates continua. While these continua may be marked by sentinel events, phases, and transitions, continuity is the persistent motif. Aging is a biological progression that occurs throughout the life span of an individual. The individual is an organism in which progressive change is seen in subcellular and cellular processes, tissue and organ structure, organ function, and organism-environment interaction.

Diseases that occur predominately in late life and are thought to have a relationship to advancing age likely represent convergence of intrinsic aging processes and organism-environment effects. Innate mechanisms, potentialities, and extrinsic forces coalesce at subcellular, cellular, tissue, and organ levels, becoming tangible in clinical condition, disorder, or disease. Cancer is cast as interaction of cellular-level environmental exposure with genetic predeterminations along with senescence—or cellular aging—processes expressed in late life. Other diseases represent different aspects of aging. Current understanding of heart failure, for example, reflects fairly sophisticated knowledge of organ-level dysfunction and its attendant systemic effects. Alzheimer's disease and other forms of dementia are explained at as yet rudimentary levels within this same paradigm. While the matrix of innate, potential, and extrinsic mechanisms remains apparent, the detail in which they are understood varies. For instance, current science shifts ostensibly time-durable explanations of cancer and aging from immune dysfunction to interwoven issues of genes, carcinogens, and immune surveillance. Complex behaviorally mediated and environmentally bound biological mechanisms remain incompletely explicated, promising advances followed by further unexplained questions.

Scientific tension arises between advancing explication of complex mechanisms in both aging and cancer and long-held averments on the nature of aging and cancer influencing what it is to be old and have cancer in our society. At a most fundamental level, embedded constructions of what it is to be old and have cancer stand invisibly behind appraisal and judgment of that state. Integrating forward-moving knowledge into socially constructed images is fraught with resistance, challenges, and transmutations. Received views are challenged, usually from different standpoints, and transmutation occurs in iterative accretion of new knowledge. That iterative accretion tends to represent ontological concerns of received views and discrete elements of legitimate knowledge as they are disseminated within and outside specific disciplines played out in a social context. Core tension in understandings of being old and having cancer exists in the social construction that emphasizes outcomes of aging—namely, functional decline and cumulative loss—juxtaposed against science that establishes aging as a process without organismal chronological commencement.

Assertion of tension in understandings of being old and having cancer emerges most often in discrimination based on chronological age or the perception of it. This discrimination is called ageism. Discrimination, while implying no particular value in or character of the word, promotes social judgment, where greater or lesser value is appraised and acted upon, but may limit individual evaluation within society. Ageism is then appraisal and action based on age as it is defined in chronological sensibilities through societal discourse. Chronological age serves as the well spring from which social discourse on aging and being old is drawn. While knowledge of aging at other levels (e.g., the cellular level) grows, integration of such knowledge has yet to transform broader social discourse. Hence chronological age is a logical reference point when age is oppugned. As a result, chronological age is the point from which issues of age and being old are discerned. Discrimination, or ageism, occurs as generally negative images of being old are situated and weighed in a particular context.

Ageism extends from social images of aging and what it means to be old in a society, ours or any other where chronological age and what is inferred from it are culturally specific (Levy 2001). Ageism can readily be described in three classes. Most prominent is probably the politically incorrect elder or "granny" bashing, an overtly negative ageism that is the most vividly prejudicial. More recently, self-stereotyping on the part of elders has come to light (Levy 1996; Levy, Ashman, and Dror 1999; Levy and Langer 1994). Self-stereotyping is perhaps a less pejorative and internalized negative ageism wherein elders judge themselves less able or deserving based on perceived social representations of their own chronological ages, yet its effects can be strikingly negative (Levy 2003). Positively intended ageism, or what I have come to call reverse parentalism, emerges far more insidiously. Fragility and incapacity are implied

by socially constructed notions of aging and being old. These characteristics beget need, especially the need for compensation and provision
of care. Compensation and care provoke thoughts of surrogacy and pa-
rental action, though the primary relationship is generally reversed in
familial situations, where a child is likely to be providing care, as it is in
professional contexts of health care delivery where clinicians are generally younger than those for whom they care. While positively intended,
compensation and care are quickly unbalanced by assumption and im-
patience. This is readily seen in the case of an adult child who, without
any supporting cultural interdiction, speaks for her parent who, while
able to speak, is judged incapable of correct sentiment in both content
and timeliness.

The inconstancy of ageism is largely determined by cultural precepts
filtered through a family's interpretation and daily life ways. The most
conspicuous example is found in imagining what constitutes appropriate
surrogacy and representation of an elder's voice for that individual who
is situated in a familial and cultural context of history, preference, and
precedent. The degree to which one must give voice or speak for one's
parent is culturally dictated and predicates a range of meanings from
respect to diminution. Cultural elements of self-stereotyping are less
easily appreciated. In part, interaction that engenders self-stereotyping
is distant from the discrimination itself. The intrapersonal nature of
self-stereotyping further complicates full comprehension of cultural
influences. Openly pejorative ageism, or granny bashing, is as overt as
parentalism but more laden with purely negative emotion. Thus I find
it more difficult to parse cultural imbrications and contemporary social
proscription. For example, what in European American stereotypes of
senility arises from cultural values placed on autonomy and self-control,
and what remains that is tied up in contemporary debate and discomfort
around tolerance for and invisibility of those perceived to be less than
fully able?

Ageism is most often apprehended in language used to convey the
discrimination at hand. Emphasis on a particular aspect or connotation
of old age engenders specific language. For example, chronological age
is most often emphasized in our society, generating concrete language
of birth dates. Chronological age typifies the notion that discrimination
can be positive or negative given contextual connotations. For example,
chronological age may be seen as a source of celebration as in a milestone birthday—especially if it exceeds expectation, as for a centenarian.
Conversely, chronological age in late life can be viewed negatively as a
point of exclusion from particular health care treatments or procedures
with the implication that proximate mortality or fragility implied by a
precise age mandates exception by age.

Using language of chronological age as opposed to biological age or age-related functional status shapes differential understandings and entails particular logical consequences. A cancer surgery, for instance, may not be offered to an older adult if chronological age is used as an eligibility criterion, whereas the surgery may be offered if organ function is the determining consideration. Less concretely, we can barely imagine what language of lived experience, that narrative notion of an individual's cumulative life experiences, or self and identity, as they pertain to capacity and motivation, might be and beget as secondary criteria in the same surgical decision. Language used to describe age and being old creates, as with any language, a set of assumptions that creates a restricted set of choices among all those possible. Deconstructing ageism requires cognizance of connectedness among language, assumptions, choice, and restriction. Language can then be used intentionally to focus on issues of greatest consequence in being old in the same way that it is used to diminish and degrade older adults.

Tension inherent in current constructions of what it means to be old and have cancer will shift as science unfolds ideas and social experience contradicts some shared images and collective understandings. However, inattention to elements of current constructions risks change that further divides rather than integrates basic, social, and applied clinical science. Interlaced biological and social science becomes more improbable as one dimension or another of the construction is given greater social weight and as dichotomies are reinforced. Emergence of the genomic era has driven an infatuation with cellular and subcellular mechanisms for disease (Hall 2003). The metaphor of errant cells preponderates, the solution for which must then be found in discovering the error itself. While cancer is clearly a process fundamentally about cellular senescence, exposure, and mutation, it is experienced as a disease at organismal and human levels and most often by older adults.

Two competing metaphors attest to the difficulty we have in approaching this realm of understanding being old and having cancer. The demographically stylized image of clichéd baby boomers driving generally positive changes in health care with the much-vaunted generational "me first" signature easily captures the public's, or at least the media's, imagination. Economic consequences entailed by the size of this generation are often supposed to explain its lasting fascination. Less visibly, the baby boomer generation offers less threatening or softer access to understanding aging and being old. As baby boomers enter the classically chronologically defined domain of being old upon reaching the age of sixty, they can be seen as old but in favorable ways—in generative family groups, employed outside the home, and physically and mentally active—that avoid fearsome, negatively perceived connotations of being

old. Though this point of access to being old is epidemiologically dissonant with incidence of several common cancers peaking around the age
of sixty, the constructed image of old age as active and attractive, and set
apart from being old and having disease, reinforces dichotomous understandings of aging and age-related disease (Jemal et al. 2005).

In an obverse metaphor, the experience of having cancer is increasingly objectified and, to a certain extent, glamorized by interplay of
charitable work to raise awareness coupled with popularized and even
celebrated images. While the public profile of breast cancer was the
first major exemplar of this metaphor of public glamour, more recently
Lance Armstrong and his survival of testicular cancer, as an icon in
popular media and private scientific funding, symbolizes embedded notions of youth, celebrity, and power in overcoming cancer. The experience of cancer in the images created around Lance Armstrong moves
past having cancer to surviving after cancer, a change not possible for
many older adults who will live with cancer as a chronic illness. This
understanding of cancer survivorship embodied by Armstrong further
reinforces characteristics—physical attractiveness, athletic power, public
celebrity—not generally associated with collective depictions of what it is
to be old in our society.

Metaphors offering activity and attractiveness oppose our collective
social notions of being old and having cancer with connotations of dysfunction, loss, and misery. Fundamental discomfort with mortality, dying,
and death seems to undergird this tension in social construction. Aging
and the proximate mortality of a finite human life span are elemental
in human existence. Within that commonality is experience unique to
the individual and particular to the life lived. General aversion to explic-
itly stated mortality is, as noted, developmentally characteristic as is the
counterbalance of a proximate personal sense of one's own mortality.
This is perfectly sensible in a biological sense where survival and pro-
creation are paramount. More abstractly, though, meaning attributed to
one's own mortality and nonfigurative anticipation of dying and death
conjure personally bound notions of suffering.

Suffering, as an extensive and intricate aspect of human existence, is
at base not something that can be evaluated from a place external to the
one who suffers. It can likely only be gauged except in the most extreme
situations (e.g., intentional torture or unrelieved physical pain). In less
extreme but no less significant situations, one person's suffering cannot
be judged by another person and thus is innately particularistic. What
constitutes suffering for one individual may not for another. In contrast
with comfort and pleasure, similarly based in an existential commonality but interpreted in individualistic preference, the place of experience
and expectation are perceptible. Suffering around mortality, dying, and

death are mediated by expectation of and aversion to these ideas and life events. Imagining what might bring mortality and lead to death then too must be symbolically avoided in human narrative.

Reflecting on what conjures suffering in being old and having cancer immediately calls forth mortality, dying, and death as being old and having cancer separately connote them. Together, the negative images attached to being old and having cancer are an existential mathematical square rather than a linguistic double negative. Each set of images makes them more negative in relation to one another. Each aspect of the construction worsens implications of dying and death abstracted in the other. The implications are derived from separately held, historically and culturally based accreted notions. Parallel moral understandings of aging well or badly in correspondence to how life has been lived are seen in the idea that the state of having cancer represents moral judgment. Modern interpretations of that moral judgment are blatantly visible in value-laden apprehensions of tobacco-use behaviors and social understandings—as opposed to biological evidence—of having cancers in which tobacco is known as a source of related carcinogens. Additionally, social constructions both of being old and of having cancer imply more proximate mortality. Culturally, cancer is still understood as a lethal disease as it shows itself variably through a history of ineffective diagnosis and arduous treatment. Combined historical, moral, and cultural forces culminate in the mathematically squared negative social construction of being old and having cancer.

Emerging science, success in treatment, and individual experience of living with, rather than dying from, cancer in late life controvert inherently negative current social constructions of being old and having cancer. Approximately half of those of any age diagnosed with cancer today go on to survive it, and many older adults diagnosed will die of a cause other than their cancer (Jemal et al. 2005). Certainly, adept critical interpretation of pertinent science and recognition of treatment outcomes has much to do with future shifts in negative images within the construction of being old and having cancer. But conversely, political priorities rooted in scientific desirability and worthiness within the received view are simultaneously derived from socially important intellectual constructions. Inverse tension results in restricting rapid change in image and all but incremental shifts in construction. More compellingly, individual narrative grounds imagined consequences of images in personal experience. Narrative then offers a point of departure for confirming or disputing collective constructions.

Through narrative, older adults who have cancer recount living with what lies within and what is marginal to socially constructed perceptions of their experience. Human narrative generally compels consideration of what is particular to the individual and extraction of what seems common across similar experiences. Furthermore, narrative offers language of experience, words used to describe it from the inside. Representations of time, event, consequence, decision, and feeling are revealed in the language used.

Health care for older adults facing cancer or other serious disease often seems organized around primary acknowledgment of time through proximate mortality and consequence of possession. Certain components of treatment and care are expropriated by clinicians and the system itself. The treatment and expectations of its efficacy are taken to be within the system. This possession then implies discernment of relative value in treatment for a particular individual, a judgment that may or may not represent ageist elements, that ties treatment itself to the ageism embedded in the social construction. That is, an older adult will generally only be offered what is deemed fitting for disease and person. The offer may be predicated on an understanding of the individual seen to have a disease or may be presented based on the disease and host characteristics of the older adult, such as chronological age. Broadly speaking, the older adult will not be entreated to reveal experience, perspective, and preference in advance of the offer, though preference is almost certainly elicited directly or indirectly (i.e., from younger family members or those who are not too ill to respond). In that asymmetry, older adults are generally left in possession of their life, though likely not their decisions about health and other instrumental aspects of that life and their cancer or other disease. Cancer and other diseases with bodily bases are viewed to be of the individual, in contrast to diseases of the mind or psyche that are still seen, despite growing cellular and molecular evidence, as being of the family. Most remarkable, perhaps, is the way in which this possession imbues language of cancer treatment. Clinically, a person treated for cancer is said to have failed therapy if the treatment was ineffective. The ascription is to the person rather than the treatment, which is the province of clinicians, and to temporal evaluation of success or failure.

Ascribing failure to the person with cancer rather than to the treatment or the clinician delivering it stems from a perspective afforded from the place of giving treatment, of wearing the mantle of clinician. Social constructions around being old and having cancer must ordinarily arise within that external perspective with attributions centered on events in that state of being that can be appreciated externally. External appraisal of attributes is based on episodic exposure through time and conveys attributes in static images that often portray extremes instead of ranges in that state of being. Social constructions can be dissected as collective images and external understandings that influence social place and labeling, and priority and choice, in the enterprise of science and health care. This dissection suggests that seeking internally mediated perspectives from those whose experience the construction delimits poses new direction.

Narrative and narrative time, as continuous rather than episodic experience, situate aims to discern meaning differently from classic analyses of socially constructed understandings. Narrative moves away from visible extremes and episodic appraisal toward reflective summary, storytelling, and continuity. Seeking narrative offers the opportunity to mark evolution in effects of dissemination and collective thought in science, health care, and society in rapidly developing issues such as being old and having cancer. Dynamic demographics and swift change in science within this domain affect socially held knowledge that may contradict or reinforce social constructions. Exploring narrative generates understanding that counterbalances evolution in which images, care, and thought become more or less irrelevant to those whose experience is wrought into that construction.

Chapter 5
Language Lessons

The experience of older adults who have cancer is likely more deeply marked by conceptual commonalities of their own language and the daily living that comprises such experience than by any discrete, scientific indicators of physiological, psychological, or social aging (Kagan 2004). In my work, three concepts that emerged from my original research in the symptom experience of older adults being treated for cancer have manifested in innumerable clinical situations and in the observation of the work of colleagues (Kagan 1994, 1997). The concepts, labeled "integrating cancer into a life mostly lived," an abstraction of the place cancer holds in the lives of older adults; "symptom stories," a representation of how older adults situate cancer and noncancer symptoms in their daily lives; and "quality of daily living," a term describing the evaluation of symptom stories and the broader illness experience within a life mostly lived (Kagan 1994, 1997), have had consistent clinical relevance in my practice and my observations of the practice of other nurses. Together, these three concepts speak to fundamental experiential aspects of living with cancer for older adults. As abstract entities, they constitute overarching psychological and social process, embodied experience, and personal appraisal of value in daily life within the experience of cancer for older adults (Kagan 1994, 1997).

In this chapter I posit that fundamental experiential aspects of cancer for older adults—and therefore nursing addressed to that experience—are abstractly represented by these three concepts. They can be employed to frame an understanding and theoretically ground care of older adults who have cancer within parameters that then echo their own experiences. Discussion of voice and power in health care for older adults and of language and consequence of ageism provides context for these concepts. After offering context, I detail the three concepts and illustrate each with clinical exemplars. I conclude the discussion with directions for new approaches to care and the translation of the concepts into care.

Dominance and power permeate health care for older adults, indeed as they may for many younger adults. Clinician dominance and power over older adults becomes more striking as complexity in care increases and negative images of aging persist (Kearney et al. 2000). Generational and social expectations of what it is to be old in any cultural context center on role, place, and voice in that society. In an abstract sense, conceptual voice represents the individual in a delineated community. It is the symbolic self in dialogue with others. In many Western societies like America, older voices may be muted or even lost in a larger social collective. Older voices, those of people judged older by social standards, are often less authoritative than younger voices, though those older voices may still be respected. Older voices are often thought to be less knowledgeable while younger voices are paradoxically accorded expert status on many issues. Further, older voices are generally heard as less clear and articulate with the vernacular notion of lost capacity in advancing age. As these impressions of older voices come together, the dominance and power of clinicians in health care over older adults is readily apparent. Clinicians are younger voices in a skilled domain. In their dominance and power lies the benevolent intent of health care wrapped in the complex knowledge of disease, treatment, and recovery.

Distance generally emerges between knowledge conveyed to the older patient and knowledge sufficient to participate meaningfully in one's own health care. Expectations for outcomes of health care are lost in that distance. Health care outcomes that are most valued in society—such as the cure or control of disease—are inherently accorded to the domain of clinicians, as the patient has little intellectual access to them. Popular understandings of the details of specific diseases and their treatment are increasingly obscure. This obscurity is echoed in the proscription of current health care where clinicians and their patients struggle under limitations of benefit and payment structures. Clinicians, not always entirely willingly, proscribe health care for their older adult patients, constrained by a system poorly matched to ageing and chronic disease. Clinicians may often view older adults' participation in health care as peripheral and direct their engagement in self-care out of necessity stemming from increasingly labyrinthine knowledge, technologies, and choices.

Embedded within issues of voice, power, and dominance in health care for older adults are discriminations made on the basis of age.[1] In America, age permeates daily dialogue and larger discourse. Age, particularly advancing age in adulthood, is omnipresent. Attempts to describe a person without reference to age in either direct or relative ways are nearly impossible. It is difficult to imagine an interpersonal world without evaluation of age. For example, one's birth date is simultaneously used in many societies as a means of identification, a point of celebration, and often—as we reach a certain age—a point of humor or even overt ridicule. The myriad aspects of age and aging in many Western societies trigger many negative or immoderate images and then entail the extremity of stereotypes (Levy and Langer 1994).

Language used in clinical discourse belies the values embedded and the directions intended in discussion of matters of age and aging. Most obviously, clinicians use language of chronological age for care every day. Many health care institutions and systems use birth date to identify patients. Age is commonly part of care protocols, as in national cancer screening recommendations that prescribe certain actions across age groups. But more insidiously, advancing age is held to mark frailty, or at least physical fragility. While chronological age can be a place of celebration in reaching a milestone birthday, it is easily be a point of discrimination when a clinical decision is predicated on chronological age as a primary criterion. Rarely is chronological age an indicator that one health care intervention is more appropriate than another or that a treatment is not worthwhile or potentially ineffective (Miller 1999; Yancik and Ries 2000). Yet clinicians oftentimes will still note that a patient "is too old" or "past the age" for a treatment like surgery or another procedure viewed as requiring youthful strength and stamina to endure. Very old chronological age elicits this reaction as often as does biological frailty that is not associated with advanced age. Rarely though is this discrimination made in the same way with a young or middle-aged adult for whom chronological age is still clinically invisible. An ageist response, though more rare with efforts to educate clinicians of all disciplines and particularly physicians, nurses, and social workers, is still more common than not. The diffusion of specialized knowledge about the effects of aging and best practices in the care of older people remains a specialty, not common knowledge.

Clinical language has yet to become clearly imbued with more keenly constructed language of biological age or functional status as labels that more adequately represent the ability and capacity of the person in body and mind (Repetto and Balducci 2002). We are increasingly able to measure discrete or proxy indicators of biological age through aspects such as organ function and functional status through physical and cognitive measures. Careful measurement allows change and response to be traced over time (Repetto and Balducci 2002). Less tangible is the idea that as innately reflective human beings we create a sense of our own being as we age and accumulate experience. Consequently, a sense of that lived experience and immingled notions of self and identity offer yet another way to represent aging and being old. This language may offer a more precise explication of the aging self than, for example, chronological age does.

No language that connotes any aspect or version of age—whether chronological age, functional status, or aging identity—befits all situations in health and social care. Yet all language implies choice: choosing to describe age and aging in a particular way and the assumption that the language chosen represents age in the most appropriate way. Language used generates action out of this choice and assumption. The worth of the language lies in its representation of age and aging within a particular context, as no set of words is ever comprehensive enough to capture all aspects of phenomena as complex as age and aging. In that worth then is the tension between choice and assumption and the restriction of what cannot be included in a chosen representation of age and aging.

Clinicians ordinarily impart specific language to describe age and aging within the context of the power and dominance they wield in health care. They choose the language of age, and older adults then respond to that language, describing themselves in the circumstance of their health care. Investigating the language that older adults use without bias imposed on them by clinicians and more broadly by society to describe age, aging, illness, and their experience constitutes a provocative reversal of power and a reordering of hierarchy. But imagine a future in which the language used by older adults frames the larger discourse of their health care and which clinicians must begin by learning their language.

The three concepts highlighted earlier in the chapter, "integrating cancer into a life mostly lived," "symptom stories," and "quality of daily living," surface as central elements of a grounded theory (Kagan 1994, 1997). These concepts distilled the language used by the older adults who informed that study of cancer and symptom experience of older adults. The language was employed to describe daily life, being treated for cancer, and effects on other aspects of life. The language, as it emerged, contrasts sharply with typical socially constructed impressions of what it is to be old and have cancer.

Most prominently, the socially mediated, all-encompassing notion of being old and having cancer is still largely one of terminal illness in late life. Society—both lay people and clinicians—still situates cancer for older adults as an end-of-life issue, drawing on social impressions of cancer as a generally lethal illness rather than a chronic illness. The chronicity of cancer treatment is outweighed by often ageist ideas that older adults are unable to withstand the rigors of cancer treatment and will therefore die of their disease. Such a stance neglects evidence that older adults are often faced with one or more diseases that are comorbid with the diagnosis of cancer and that older adults may in fact tolerate some facets of cancer treatment with less distress than their younger counterparts (Kagan 2004). Finally, the construction of cancer as a terminal illness avoids the temporal and developmental understanding of one's own mortality.

Older adults, in the original grounded theory, conveyed their understanding that death was a proximate reality given their relatively advanced ages (Kagan 1994). The informants were uniform in their depiction of acknowledging that they had lived most of their natural life span. Cancer was portrayed as one element of health and illness in life but was not a central focus for many. Hence, the concept "integrating cancer into a life mostly lived" captures the interconnection of advancing age, understanding one's life, and experiencing cancer.

The concept of "symptom stories," simply stated, stands opposite the clinically laden term *symptom management* as the standard for understanding and ameliorating symptoms of cancer or of comorbid disease and side effects of biomedical treatment. Symptom management implies an external process of direction and intervention to achieve success. It also connotes a businesslike and organized focus on the symptoms. Conversely, older adults commonly experience a multitude of embodied physical and psychological sensations that may be symptoms or side effects of one or more illnesses, treatments, or both (Kagan 2004). Older adults then live day to day with this array of symptoms and side effects. The sensations, attributed causes, perceived meanings, acceptable treatments, and evaluated outcomes spiral together to create an encompassing experience. Elements of the experience fall within the realm of health care, for example, in pharmacological or behavioral intervention, to ameliorate a symptom. Other elements do not, as is often seen in the experience of patients whose symptom experience exceeds expectations for reasons of personal meaning and valuation. Hence the complexity of symptom management that grows with advancing age and the cumulative experience of one's body and its responses is better captured by the term *symptom stories.*

The third concept, "quality of daily living," is perhaps most at odds with the received view of valuing the effects of health care and evaluation of health and illness experience in the broader picture of an individual's life (Kagan 2004). Quality of life is the universally employed and deeply embedded representation of the global outcome most sought after—surviving disease, cancer in this case, is a character of acceptable function, ability, and pleasure. Quality of life is addressed in a vast theoretical, quantitative, and—to a lesser degree—qualitative literature (Donaldson 2004). It is the impetus for detailed questionnaires or tools aimed at measuring this concept in precisely defined groups of patients. Most important, quality of life is a fundamental phrase in the clinical argot of clinicians, patients, and the lay public alike.

When measured by most tools used in clinical care, quality of life is appraised in retrospect via questions determined by those who ask—not those who answer—to be important aspects of quality. Popular tools may ask about work and play, about mundane activities such as shopping for food, and presence of physical symptoms and mood disturbance over a period of a few weeks. Most often such questions are posed in a youth-centered fashion that assumes work outside the home and other characteristics of daily life that may be more varied with advancing age. The retrospective time frame asks for general appraisal and cannot track daily change. These questions also presume that individual variation will recede against the collective value of commonplace activity balanced against frequent symptoms. In a broad sense, the recession of incidental individual variation is true and in certain ways important. Nonetheless, losing variation in predetermined questions and time frames entails diminished specificity and precision that may be clinically significant.

Older adults who have cancer most commonly use language in the present tense to evaluate the quality they find in their lives. And they employ comparative language to frame their description in the sense of the immediate. Retrospective appraisal is less often used and is less resonant. For example, older adults may say, "Today is better than yesterday" or "This morning was not good, but this afternoon is going well." This approach enables older adults to review their present experience and reflect discrete feelings of lesser or greater quality. The present tense and immediate description frame relative value and change while comparison evaluates what is possible and desirable for that person, rather than what is normative or standard. The present, immediate, comparative language of evaluation is constituted in "quality of daily living." The concept also avoids confounding global satisfaction with one's life with evaluation of its daily quality. While global satisfaction and daily quality are surely linked, they are also distinct ideas.

In this section, I describe each of the three concepts with reference to the grounded theory perspective in which they were developed and the clinical exemplars that illuminate them. The conceptual characteristics and theoretical place of each is detailed with reference to how it contributes to understanding the experience of older adults who have cancer. Last, I explore implications for clinical care and inquiry.

"Integrating cancer into a life mostly lived," in the terminology of grounded theory, is a core concept. As such, it unifies the concepts that compose the grounded theory and foretells its character and nature. In terms of grounded theory, "integrating cancer into a life mostly lived" is a type of concept called a basic psychological process. That basic psychological process offers a representation of what it is to be old and have cancer through the embodied experience of knowing the cancer through symptoms and side effects. This concept, then, has several inherent qualities. It is specific to older adults who appraise their sense of a proximate mortality. It speaks to a focus on a daily life wider than that centered on health care interactions and experiences. It understands experiences and the process of having cancer as an older adult through its embodiment.

Finally, at a level of intricate, socially created and shared meaning, "integrating cancer into a life mostly lived" offers an alternative to the common metaphor for cancer. Most prominently in American understanding, war is the metaphor for cancer experience. This metaphor is most simply predicated on youth, focused exclusively on the cancer, and aimed at success in survival. Battles against cancer implied by the metaphor are won or lost, culminating in victory or defeat vis-à-vis the disease itself.[2] The young generally possess the physical vigor and undivided focus necessary for waging war. The implicit immortality that is necessary for battles of youth hopes to proclaim absolute victory, as loss suggests mortality.

Battles are certainly not exclusive to youth, however, and the language of it pervades descriptions of disease and care. In Chapter 1, Mrs. Eck eloquently describes battling cancer in a subtly different form. Her story connotes that the war was waged as much against a system refractory to her needs as against the pancreatic cancer that necessitated her interaction with it. Her realism tempers her aims and composes the aims of battle in relation to that which is desired and achievable: time with family, function, and comfort. Mrs. Eck's story is imbued with her own sense of more proximate but not immediate mortality, balanced against enjoyment and desire for life. She represents the gradual accession to a personal mortality and deep understanding that one's life is not limitless that normally is concomitant with advancing age and personal emotional development. The delicate tension, between desiring one's life and knowing the propinquity of one's death that proceeds as life is lived, reduces the resonance of the metaphor of war and its denoted aim of survival for older adults who have cancer.

Integration is the obverse of the singular focus in the war metaphor, providing a wider range for age, gender, power, and preference. The integration central to "cancer in a life mostly lived" further implies that survival alone within the frame of proximate mortality is an insufficient metric for success. Individual interpretation of terms for success stems from the consequent concept of quality of daily living inside the umbrella of integration.

"Integrating cancer into a life mostly lived" restructures foundations on which images of being old and having cancer are constructed. It conceptually situates cancer in the context of late life rather than death. Older adults give voice to their lives and the meaning cancer holds in the process of daily activities. This placement enables greater focus on patterns established over a lifetime. As a result, cancer becomes less an anomalous disturbance that threatens death and more an experience in a range of health and illness over a life course. Further, "integrating cancer into a life mostly lived" emphasizes functional status through its focus on daily life. This emphasis is in keeping with principles of generally understood gerontological care as well. The foundational shift achieved by "integrating cancer into a life mostly lived" then frames clinical care with older adults who have cancer, encompassing the experience of cancer, other illnesses, and life preferences. Most important in clinical care, the larger frame and central focus on the older adult allows open goal setting and facilitates treatment appropriate to the person.

"Symptom stories" might represent the most clinically and personally practical concept emerging from this analysis of older adults' experience of cancer and cancer treatment. Symptom stories are the direct personal temporal narrative of the embodied experience of changing sensations, responses, meanings, actions, and outcomes perceived as connected to the cancer and its treatment. In typical health care discourse, that sequence is labeled as "symptom" or "side effect." Once labeled, a particular symptom or side effect is attributed to cancer, coexisting illness, cancer treatment, or therapy for those other illnesses. The process of managing the symptom or side effect is then divided. Symptom management becomes the purview of clinicians while the response to symptoms remains the domain of the patient. A power gradient surfaces in ownership, control, and intervention. Older adults with cancer are more likely to tell a more intricate story of interaction, relationship, meaning, and comfort around symptoms and side effects. Intervention may be embedded in seemingly small choices, patterns, or preferences predicated in previously acquired self knowledge. There may be little differentiation among symptoms and side effects of cancer and comorbid illness, in contrast to typical clinical approaches that seek to differentiate cause and effect to understand and treat each alone.

The symptom story itself is told in retrospect, as a story. Past and current experiences perceived by the older person who tells the story to have bearing on the symptom of present focus create the context and background. The story is iterative, told in a cycle of changed sensation or feeling, evaluated discomfort or distress, and compared previous experience followed by action taken and effect appraised against a leveled expectation of reduced discomfort or distress. This iterative cycle can be repeated over time as the story is told in retrospect and remains unresolved and incomplete at the time of the telling, or it can be resolved and told completely in the past as a closed experience. Hence symptom stories are most readily grouped by their resolution; they are either *incomplete*, using past experience and other resources in the aim of expected relief, or *complete*, ready to be drawn into future symptom experience as a fund of knowledge about response and relief.

Symptom stories function to fit symptoms into a basic psychological process that characterizes this grounded theory. The fit is achieved as older adults who have cancer select personal strategies from their previous experience with illness or even from caregiving for ill family members along with recommendations from clinicians, finding balance in their own embodied knowledge and the information supplied to them. Symptom stories are built through iterations of reflection on knowledge and experience and actions based in that reflection. As they are built, tension and activity are easily seen as the means through which symptom stories take shape.

In a follow-up study to the original grounded theory (Kagan 1994), patients and their clinicians represented symptom stories differentially if symptom management is taken as the clinician view of symptom stories. Patients emphasized dialogue with clinicians and others, revealing a process centered on relationships. A man in his seventies who had been diagnosed with several primary cancers in his lifetime said: "Compassion [that's what is important in symptom management and care]—some of them [doctors and nurses] treat patients like idiots." His symptom stories, like those of so many of my patients, seemed predicated on social interaction and developing relationships with clinicians to underpin further work together. In this part of the process, older adults appear to rely on past illness experience as a source of knowledge that comes near to bodily wisdom.

Clinicians spoke of creating a management process for patients. Management was proscribed and separated from relationship. A medical oncologist noted: "One of the aspects of my medical style is to . . . try to be light and—not have very weighty conversations [unless they are necessary]." He went on to say: "And part of it is that I think I want them to feel comfortable and agree [with the plan]." Creation of symptom management involves outlining expectations of what to feel and what to call symptoms or side effects, though this seems to be more pronounced with side effects where therapies are defined in part by a profile of attributed side effects. Management interventions were then based on those predetermined expectations, setting up potential disruption if expectations were exceeded and possible relief if they were not met.

Plotting symptom stories is easily accomplished and likely clinically useful. Clinicians can uncover past illness experience and encourage reflection on, and use of, them in the present experience of cancer. The iterative, rather abstract character of symptom stories highlights that chronicity plus the very practical degree to which strategies work and expectations of relief are met or managed determines whether the story itself is complete or incomplete. Using this simple mechanism for understanding overcomes the common clinical tension that arises in the markedly different ways that patients and clinicians approach symptoms and side effects. Patients use life experiences to frame expectations of how symptoms might feel and guide their own management toward "what works" for them based on their own experience along with information provided by clinicians. Clinicians may not elicit this information and see symptom management as something they prescribe through therapeutic intervention alone.

The final concept, "quality of daily living," structures valuation within "integrating cancer into a life mostly lived." As a temporally framed, present-focused but retrospectively achieved metric, it highlights the centrality of daily function and preferred activities. "Quality of daily living" conceptually outlines personal, intrinsic markers of quality rather than relying solely on externally set standards for function and activities selected by a researcher or other external authority and not the person whose life is being measured. The evaluation of "quality of daily living" emphasizes abilities to interact as an endpoint of function and activity, as in primary familial or social relationships, and comfort, as in relief from the discomfort and distress of physical and psychological symptoms. "Quality of daily living" is then personally evaluative. Each older adult serves as her or his own "control" in the terminology of research, setting baseline expectations and a criterion against which to judge change. Such a progressive baseline stands opposite the usual understanding of a static, generic baseline established in typical measurement of quality of life. Ultimately, "quality of daily living" becomes a progressive and contextual measurement of "what's good for me now" that reflects how expectations, goals, and desires can change over the course of an illness as an individual accumulates experiences and lives over that time in the context of a life mostly lived.

In clinical care, "quality of daily living" can balance the clinician-patient-family relationship as it uses a personal metric for evaluation and allows and accounts for change over time. Further, it lends itself to decision making in these conceptual characteristics as it avoids global, distant evaluation directed by many current measures of quality of life. "Quality of daily living" reframes a clinically directed evaluation toward one centered on the individual, using criteria that hold personal meaning. It resonates with what language clinicians hear from their patients in everyday dialogue about daily life.

Language is a tool that undergirds most human interactions, both personal and professional. It is deeply embedded in our lives, immediately available and familiar, and visible most when it is absent. Language speaks of and to what is most obvious and concrete in our daily lives as much as to what is most ephemeral and intangible in how we value our lives. Language in the case of older adults who have cancer easily represents personal interpretations of identity, family, culture, and care if we listen closely to it. In whatever society and culture in which nursing provides care, specific reflection on language is probably underestimated as a means to improve that care.

The three concepts discussed here—"integrating cancer into a life mostly lived," "symptom stories," and "quality of daily living"—arose from inquiry into the experience of cancer and cancer symptoms for older adults and offer a different perspective on aspects of being old and having cancer. This perspective is one that diverges from the received view of being old and having cancer as sad terminus, disconnected from the life a person has lead before cancer. Admittedly, this perspective accentuates advantages of being old and having cancer through a focus on living as opposed to previous emphases on terminal illness and impending death. Further, it conceptually outlines the role and placement of the experience of cancer in older adults' lives and reveals facets of the clinician-patient relationship, and perhaps other relationships as well. As an alternative view, however, these concepts in particular highlight gaps in care posed by the mismatch among the desires and experience of older adults who have cancer, current care, and available evidence to guide future care.

These three concepts have clear conceptual implications for relationships in care. The language that older adults use to describe their experience of cancer has less to do with their age and more to do with who they are as individuals. These concepts each explain and frame elements of relationships that older people with cancer may have with clinicians, family, and friends. Using such ideas suggests new ways to balance expectations, particularly those of clinicians, and offer new possibilities for understanding and evaluation. Indeed, their application posits that it is possible and practical to theoretically inform practical, daily care.

Chapter 6
Aesthetics of Being and Having

What it means to be old and have cancer is ultimately a very individual matter, a personal experience of self—a persona of identity, embodiment, and relationships in daily life. It is out of such experiences that collective sensibilities emerge and social thought on the state of being old and having cancer extends. The remnants of our society's Protestant origins that I discussed earlier, in order to frame the modern stories of Mrs. Eck, Mr. Napolitano, and Mr. Cahn, remind us of a time when cancer could not be understood in any dimension as a biological phenomenon and was exclusively a moral and social domain. In our society's history, early received views of cancer very much revolved around moral existence and the value of personal comportment. The moral rectitude of one's life emerged to a certain degree through a composite aesthetic of aging and disease. Belief held that a moral life resulted in a pleasant, or even beautiful, countenance, and could be seen in good and pure health. An immoral life, poorly lived, was thought to shape an ugly physiognomy and often to result in diseases like cancer.

Remaining elements of those religious, cultural, and social forces that intertwined cancer and morality into a historical aesthetic of disease still in part shape our current understandings of and meaning attributed to the state of being old and having cancer. However, historically embedded understandings are compounded now by rapid shifts in the cancer treatment paradigm. These shifts and changes in treatment imbue our discourse on aging and cancer with nuances that twist historically mediated ideas. Social understanding tends to lag behind advances in treatment as experience of them diffuses through discourse. Cancer treatments that may have been, not many years ago, rudimentary and ineffective now sometimes risk being perceived as radical and overreaching as we struggle to comprehend the social meaning of the science they employ. The tension between the capacity to target cancer biology and the desire to preserve aesthetic notions of personhood is often central to this struggle. Breast cancer is the most available example of this progression. Radical surgical mastectomy and, later, cobalt radiation offered a cure for breast cancer. That cure generally came with extreme distortion of the breast, torso, and hence a woman's image of herself. Current therapies aim for conservation of the breast and integration of the self even with chronic—recurrent or metastatic—disease. Clinicians are deeply aware of the threat that disfigurement and dysfunction present to the self, identity, and patterns of daily life. Similarly, social awareness of breast cancer is very high, and the old, embedded image of a woman suffering from a disfiguring and likely lethal disease is being transformed into one of a woman living with a disease that may in fact be invisible to the public eye, involving small scars or temporary side effects such as hair loss. Impact on her personal and public aesthetic is considerably changed and certainly less visible; however, I might argue that although we have changed the aesthetic of breast cancer, we cannot erase aesthetic alterations entirely. Cancer, as a disease with very real contemporary social dimensions, surely changes private and public aesthetic understandings of what it is to be human. Shifts in the treatment paradigm have diminished and changed the impact of breast cancer on women's private and public aesthetic. We have likely substituted some aspects of the aesthetic for others, yet the aesthetic dimensions persist. Where missing breasts were once paradigmatic, alopecia—hair loss—and other less characteristic byproducts of treatment are now paramount.

Aging and being old adds another dimension to the aesthetic of the self with cancer. The self that emerges as one ages integrates elements of daily life and identity, particularly influenced by embodiment of abilities and capacities that are physical, cognitive, and emotional. The experience of living in an aging body accumulates over time, barring acute changes or catastrophic events, so that aged embodiment is most often very gradual and situated in knowing oneself over time. The existential state of being—young, old, man, woman—and having—cancer—is singularly and remarkably individual and iterative. It is of the self in the most personal and fundamentally human sense and yet, because existence is in the context of others, always tinged by social influences and interaction. It is also cumulative and continually shifting with sensation, experience, perception, and interpretation. The state of being and having imparted by being old and having cancer necessarily shapes and hones the personal aesthetic held by any individual.

Cancer, like other serious and chronic diseases, alters embodiment with often sharp changes in ability and capacity. Such changes may be temporary or permanent, acute or insidious. Cancer and its treatment commonly generate distinct and dramatic shifts in embodiment through the illness experience that, because treatment may be arduous and the effects of disease considerable, result in lost physical condition, limited abilities, and changed capacities. Surgery and other treatments such as chemotherapy and radiation may reshape the body in large or small ways, permanently or temporarily. Even seemingly small alterations can generate profound emotional reactions, arising in any facet of the experience, that reflexively chafe self and identity. Younger people seem to react differently than older people to the experience of cancer. What may be significant at one age seems different or differentially important at another. Physical, functional, and experiential alterations that attend cancer and cancer treatment combine with the personal and social import of what it means to have cancer. The combination marks the experience of being old and having cancer as uniquely individual, being in and of the aged body and self while being socially and personally significant, as personal interpretation melds with social imaginings. The individual significance in the experience of being old and having cancer then reflects inwardly on identity and outwardly on interaction. Changes in how the individual appears and functions influence that significance.

Being and having is then, in the context of old age and cancer, elementally aesthetic in some sense. We immediately imagine the appearance, the aesthetic, of what it is to have cancer. The state of being old and having cancer, with its consequent issues of social perception, warrants detailed illustration. Representative cases can dissect images—both familiar and unfamiliar—to address how socially shared ideas influence understanding of what it is to be old and have cancer. For example, in my practice, I work with many older adults who have cancers of the mouth or throat or of the skin of the head and neck. These cancers are less common than other, better-known diseases such as breast, prostate, or colorectal cancer, the four most common cancers among older adults in the United States (Jemal et al. 2005). However, like these more common cancers, cancers of the head and neck affect mostly older adults (Jemal et al. 2005). Unlike breast, colorectal, lung, or prostate cancers, the anatomy affected by cancers of the head and neck is both visible and far less forgiving than the elastic anatomy of the breast or colon, for example, and thus head and neck cancers are aesthetically unlike these more common cancers. Individuals diagnosed with head and neck cancers may be treated with surgery, though chemotherapy and radiation are increasingly useful. Surgery commonly involves reconstruction of the affected anatomy to attempt restoration of aesthetics and function. These treatments, though difficult to undergo, clearly yield better function and quality of life than did earlier regimens of radical surgery and intensive radiation.

Head and neck cancers are emblematic of so many issues that imbue the experience of being old and having cancer with unique and intricate social import. Even with better anatomical preservation with improved treatment protocols, older people with head and neck cancers are at risk of some disfigurement and dysfunction. That risk of readily apparent change in a person's appearance and publicly held personal aesthetic distinguishes cancers of the head and neck from other cancers where the anatomy is more forgiving and is not publicly visible. Further, the functional and aesthetic changes brought about by head and neck cancers can mimic loss of function often associated with old age: loss of articulate speech, safe swallowing, and unrestricted vision. Such functional decline and loss are easily apprehended and provoke anxiety, given the centrally human nature of activities like breathing, speaking, and eating, along with immutably individual expressions of voice and affection seen in a word or a kiss. Within this frame, I argue for understanding interrelationships among advancing age and cancer to understand the aesthetics as a primary influence on social understanding of what it means to be old and have cancer. Head and neck cancers, by virtue of risks for visible and sometimes aversive disfigurement, serve as exemplars of paradoxical social invisibility emerging from aesthetic aspects of being old and having cancer.

Head and neck cancers reveal themselves in overt, public ways not generally seen in other diseases. Lung cancer, a disease that often shares the carcinogenetic effects of tobacco use with some head and neck cancers, may be nearly invisible until it is extremely advanced. It engenders a variety of externally apprehended symptoms such as weight loss, perpetual cough, shortness of breath, and disabling pain. Breast cancer less and less often alters the anatomy with organ conserving treatment. Prostate cancer often threatens functions even more intimate than that of the breast: urinary continence and sexual potency. While the effects of incontinence and impotence are generally devastating to identity, the experience is extremely private—the popularity of advertisements and celebrity spokesmen for erectile dysfunction not withstanding. In prostate cancer, as with breast cancer, the altered aesthetic is then publicly invisible, and the dysfunction is generally hidden from all but in the most intimate relationships. Likewise with colorectal cancer, tangible aesthetic implications revolve around an abdominal scar, skin changes with radiation or chemotherapy, and possibly an ostomy or diversion of the bowel to the skin's surface, all of which may be concealed from public view. Functional changes in the bowel, though they can occur as a result of colorectal cancer and its treatment, are again intimate in nature. Compared with head and neck cancers, lung, breast, prostate, and colorectal cancers carry a privacy that shapes their social imagining. Privacy ensures that a different set of sociocultural elements are played out. Taboos associated with the intimate functions apply while, conversely, head and neck cancers generate publicly mediated appraisal and the stigma associated with response to altered faces and public functions using speech and swallowing.

The experience of having a cancer of the head and neck is commonly constructed around a central repugnant image characterized by social invisibility and aversion. The stereotypical person with head and neck cancer is an old man who is often seen as unworthy of treatment because of his advanced age combined with long-time abuse of tobacco and alcohol. This negatively skewed image echoes early American, largely European Protestant historical implications of the life lived well or badly (Cole 1992). In this ethos, the badly lived, immoral life was manifest in visitation of physical and mental ills in late life (Cole 1992). Variance from the stereotype further reveals the nature of visibility within cancer experienced in late life. For example, younger women who eschew tobacco and alcohol or other people who possess characteristics that identify them as less morally deviant than the stereotype connotes confound moral elements of the aesthetic interpretation for head and neck cancer that harkens back to historical understandings of disease. How are these individuals to be understood in contrast to those who fit the stereotype of belief that they in some part have incurred disease through behavior read as immoral? The conflict between social image, stereotype, and the reality experienced by individuals who have a specific cancer—such as this case in head and neck cancer or men with breast cancer—may be dissected at larger social levels to understand forces that impinge upon the development of socially shared understandings and discourse.

Breast cancer is a prime example of a cancer that, having been peculiarly taboo in social discourse, has become a publicly acceptable and aesthetically visible malignancy. As breast cancer has become more visible to the public, political activism, charity events, celebrity pronouncements, and mass media coverage have iteratively shifted its constructed image. The dissemination of the color pink from the original awareness ribbon to almost any product one can imagine is testament to the changed social understanding of breast cancer and to the success of a public campaign in shaping that understanding. Fundamentally, the public campaign created images that played on prevalence and conjured social acceptability and even prestige to overcome taboo and aversion, creating remarkable attractiveness and activism. This is a paradigm that offers a strong counterpoint to that of head and neck cancers.

There is much less social activism for and awareness of head and neck cancers than for breast cancer. Perhaps this relative obscurity stems from the number of people affected by breast cancer as opposed to head and neck cancers. Though, to be fair, while breast cancer is a more common disease that should in some ways have a larger societal footprint, the experience of having head and neck cancer is no less deserving given less optimal survival and more pervasive possible ramifications in function. Nonetheless, people do not generally volunteer to march for throat cancer or oral cancer as they do for breast cancer—there is not the same cachet perhaps. Increasingly, much activism happens in organized support groups or on the Internet. Groups such as WebWhispers Nu-Voice Club and Support for People with Oral and Head and Neck Cancer (SPOHNC) all have easily accessed Web sites, and many have associated chat rooms, electronic mailing lists, and other electronic communication streams.[1] Parallel to the breast cancer advocacy movement, SPOHNC now markets oral and head and neck cancer awareness ribbon pins. The red and cream stripes are not as omnipresent as breast cancer pink, but then these pins are new on the awareness scene. Will there be a time when the public awareness campaign promoted by SPOHNC will have achieved the transformation of social thought to that surrounding breast cancer today?

Paradoxically, people who have head and neck cancer, their treatment, and the research that supports it have been *socially* invisible despite the actual visibility of the anatomy and function affected. Rarity of the disease, social images and hyperbolic stereotype, and even the stigmata of visibly disfiguring cancers and treatments coalesce to condition aversion in interaction and discourse. Head and neck cancer then sets up a paradigm in which we can see a conundrum of competing and often divergent or even opposing social images. These conflicting images and understandings represent what it is to have cancer in the context of a particular life. The conundrum may be overtly considered in actual practice, as for example in a tumor board discussion—an academic debate of the merits of specific treatments for particular patients. In such a discussion, the influence of social images and shared understandings is evident. For example, the manner in which disfiguring surgeries and possible reconstructions of form and perhaps function are discussed in relation to a specific patient may reveal consideration of age or gender. The case of a young patient whose physical condition would be characterized as youthfully strong and whose life is perceived as yet to be lived may be played out in discussion of aggressive treatments with risk of loss of form or function against recovery time and potential to achieve meaningful rehabilitation. An older person who may be perceived as constitutionally fragile and nearing the end of his natural life may be discussed with an eye toward conservative therapies that would aim at conservation. Within that aim of conservation, what is generally termed quality of life and a global sense that the human cost of the treatment and the recovery required were acceptable in the context of the years of life left remaining would be considered. Such detailed clinical conversations not withstanding, synthesis of the way in which complex and nuanced construction of age and cancer is notably absent from more abstract intellectual discourse.

Surgery is a common treatment or part of a treatment plan in many cases for both cancers of the breast and of the head and neck. Thus examination of surgical decisions in the contrasting cases of these cancers can further reveal aspects of the aesthetics of being old and having cancer. Reconstruction of the surgical defect is now more commonly considered part of any viable treatment plans with an aim of restoring form and function to the greatest extent possible. So, for instance, as patients seek treatment of head and neck cancer, they expect functional and aesthetic outcomes for appearance, speech, and swallowing. These desires then entail some form of reconstruction if surgery is involved and rehabilitation when radiation and chemotherapy are used. Clinicians must then strive to understand the patients' own images and identity, and their maintenance and refinement over the life course, as the meaning of cancer is confronted. The exploration of the interaction between patient and surgeon as well as other clinicians raises the question of whose image of the patient will be reconstructed within this interplay of concerns and how age and, secondarily, gender play out in addressing it.

The expectations with which a person who becomes the patient enters the cancer reconstruction process are complex. Public and private identity and social role are inherently bound to the cancer diagnosis. When a person diagnosed with head and neck cancer approaches treatment, many choices and distinct limitations become prominent. A range of possibilities exists, dependent to a certain extent on prior knowledge, advocacy, and commitment, and then to access, and, finally, to exploration and education to review available options. Over the past three decades, more reconstructive options have become possible. Over the past fifteen years in particular, more widespread surgical technologies such as microvascular techniques have become available, and anesthesia techniques have allowed older patients to undergo these increasingly complex procedures (Olson and Shedd 1978; Bridger, O'Brien, and Lee 1994). There are now reconstructive options available that—while they do not enhance survival—do contribute to quality of daily living through restoration of function and appearance, making treatment decision and action all the more intricate.

Similarly, women diagnosed with breast cancer now routinely seek breast reconstruction if breast conservation is not an option. Women invest in their breasts aspects of their private identities that are unlike the public elements of identity seen in facial aesthetics. The image of the breast itself has been constructed of social, sexual, and biological aesthetic elements. Reconstruction may offer some maintenance of a personal aesthetic, only a component of which is somewhat public.

Conversely, as a woman integrates her breast cancer into her identity, reconstruction may be less attractive, depending on generation and other personal, familial, and cultural preferences and may then be avoided as an option. The importance of the breast may be diminished after menopause or for other reasons and concerns about appearance may be mediated by prosthetic breasts and brassieres, outweighing surgical options.

In contrast to breast cancer, the head and neck, and most precisely the face and voice, are a most public representation of personhood and identity. Thus choices about reconstruction may feel less fungible when compared against rehabilitation with nonsurgical means. Public aspects of identity and aesthetics of the human face and—though less so—the neck are complicated by functions performed using involved anatomy. In many ways, then, the case of head and neck cancer demands reconstruction where it is necessary to maintain public identity and a personal aesthetic. In addition to being the most readily apprehended element of public identity, the face also often conveys some of the most intimate or private nonverbal behavior and communication. Expressions of emotion, as in kissing a child or parent, and enjoying sensual experiences, as in kissing a sexual partner, or eating a favorite and much relished meal imbue the anatomy of the face with the most human capacity. Restoration of these functions may be perceived as consonant with the quality of daily living.

Aesthetics of aging are of increasing interest in our society as we confront evolving social roles for older people and adherent matters of changing form—the aged body—and function. The aesthetics of having a disease and being ill are less engaging and acceptable, however, and therefore more difficult to apprehend. Popular culture and history further complicate perception of reconstruction and restoration of form if not function. Specifically, we think of cosmetics and the ability to camouflage for aesthetic purposes as well prototypical notions of plastic surgery as the province of women, particularly those who are older and affluent enough to afford discretionary purchases. However, the roots of modern plastic surgery in reconstructing casualties of war create a contemporary, socially prescribed schema in which men and gender in general, and indeed cancer itself with its overlying metaphors of war, are intriguingly situated (Haiken 1994, 2000). Wartime casualties often involve trauma to the head and neck. This trauma can mimic head and neck cancer and its surgical treatment. Prosthetics and masks used to camouflage neurological and head and neck cancers that affect the eyes or the nose recall the masks used to cover disfigurement from wartime casualties. The recollection of war in head and neck cancer, at least, then recalls larger metaphors of the war on cancer and makes approaching reconstruction and rehabilitation with prosthetics and camouflage in cancer less gendered and perhaps perceived as less frivolous in social discourse.

Cancer is tightly bound to war in our shared social understandings and reveals a great deal about how cancer is understood outside the context of specific diagnoses or human characteristics such as age. War, as a metaphor, divulges how fraught with risk cancer is understood to be in our society. Most fundamentally, there is risk of loss. While death is most often the risk represented in social discourse around cancer, risk of loss of form and function is also present but less often explored. Proclaiming war on cancer mandates engagement in the battle for the individual. Yet the risk of engagement is distanced in society where forward movement in the battle and in the war overall is gauged in statistics, numbers that reflect elements of the individuals but not the individuals themselves. The risk of engagement in this war is far more personal and specific for individuals. Cancer threatens embodiment. Cancer fundamentally distorts anatomy, visible or not, as it grows and invades surrounding tissue. In fact, the invasive character of cancer is remarkably aligned with the social understanding of it, even associated with the stigma connoted by cancer. Its treatment further disfigures in various ways and to various extents. That treatment may be essentially invisible and functionally recoverable as with an operation that preserves the organ affected, such as a lumpectomy in breast cancer. Or it may be highly visible and functionally life altering as in laryngectomy, removal of the voice box, for advanced cancer of the larynx. In laryngectomy, essential human functions are profoundly altered. The windpipe is diverted to exit the skin at the base of the neck so that breathing is then separated from the mouth and from functions like swallowing. Vocal capacity is lost until restored with a prosthetic sound-producing device such as a hand-held electro-larynx or more recent innovations such as a prosthetic valve that connects the windpipe and the esophagus, or food pipe, that makes use of swallowed air. Lumpectomy or laryngectomy, the aesthetics of cancer at any age are then a matter of form and function in human action and interaction. The matter of form and function is lasting too and influences life with cancer over time. The cancer and its treatment result in both temporary and permanent changes as well as alteration of the individual's perspective through experience. In this manner, the experience of cancer transcends the embedded notion of mere survival—beating the odds to live in the face a lethal prognosis—to become one of meeting long-term changes and chronic challenges with desires to achieve a certain quality in daily life.

Frequently, patients of all ages and both sexes seek the most aggressive treatment available, while desiring survival with functional aesthetic outcomes rather than merely adopting the fatalistic stance of "just lucky to be alive." They balance the multiple risks and potential losses of cancer against one another in the context of their lives. The simplistic balance of being alive or facing death diminishes the detail and consequence of treatment decisions. Older women and men present some of the greatest technical challenges to completing cancer treatment and inherent side effects given their larger likelihood of declining functional reserve compounded by physical fragility or coexisting diseases. Paradoxically, younger patients often represent more complex challenges in decision making to clinicians, who may feel responsible for finding some acceptable point in balancing successful treatment with socially acceptable aesthetic and functional morbidity. The influence of age and gender may make interpretation of available options more intricate for the clinician.

The question of whose image is to be reconstructed or even rehabilitated is rarely uncovered in clinical interviews and even more rarely fully addressed in intellectual discourse. A complex interaction ensues from considerations of the person—including age and gender, the disease and its treatment options and relevant prognoses, along with a host of more situational factors that vary from desire for and access to care to the health care resources and expertise available to any given patient. Even very personal and temporal concerns such as the objectification of a woman's beauty or the neglect of a man's aesthetic desires may arise. The context of being old in an aging society further complicates the interaction. Societal impressions that women are more vain and desirous of aesthetic results than men and that the old are less vain and less concerned with appearance than the young may work to unwitting ends. These impressions may play out as clinicians offer options they perceive as socially appropriate as well as surgically possible, while patients may struggle with an entirely different set of expectations. Conversely, as individuals present their expectations as patients, they may misunderstand the options available and the choices they face. What might be an interaction may end up as parallel monologues as social and individual understandings reveal themselves.

Consider again the image of the stereotyped individual with head and neck cancer. This stereotype highlights that the relatively low incidence of head and neck cancer, limitations and morbidity of treatment, and the risk of unappealing aesthetic outcome and functional loss work against each other paradoxically to make patients appallingly invisible and sometimes shatteringly visible in society. This aversive visibility creates the conundrum of making these patients, through that very aversion, invisible and objects to ignore. Society and even caregivers frequently view these typical patients as unworthy because of the manner in which they live their lives. At the same time, there is no room in that social construction for people who do not fit that typical image. Women of any age who have any number of cancers may find it particularly difficult to achieve an aesthetic functional outcome they and society will find acceptable. The more visible and stigmatizing the cancer, the more difficult the desired outcome may be to achieve. Deconstruction of these social forces is necessary as we come to acknowledge that issues of age and gender become paramount when we propose to treat individuals and repair damage to both aesthetic form and function.

When as a society we contend with the shifting understandings and evolving meaning attached to what it means to be old and have cancer in our society today, age and gender and other more mutable characteristics become paramount as we ask, "Are we reconstructing the patient as person or a socially constructed image of the patient?" Is there a new aesthetic being created, one cut and pasted out of age and cancer as a socially constructed disease with ever-expanding and refined health care technologies, shifting gender roles, and an aging society? The delineation of an aesthetic in cancer is a prerequisite to better understanding the quality of individual experience and clinical results and to investigate further what it means to be old and have cancer in our society today.

Epilogue
Not a Denial of the Fact of Death, a Denial of Death Now

People—enthrallingly, I think—exist in a space that merges inner identity and personal aesthetic with socially perceived knowing. As much as we comprehend ourselves and our own existence, we are known by others, especially those who love us. The dialectical nature of being in and through knowing oneself and being known by others accretes as we age. Our lives become almost labyrinthine as we pass through decades of daily life with relationships and events that mark them. This layering of experience shapes identity, knowing, and a composite aesthetic, a sense of ourselves as physically embodied beings who function in context and environment and, in that meld of existence and action, are beautiful. What precisely is found beautiful and how it is valued may be infinitely deliberated. Nonetheless, a sense of a generalized aesthetic incorporating human form and function as well as age and gender is more easily grasped. Full appreciation of the state of being old and having cancer then includes, as I have argued, its social images and shared understandings as well as its dialectically achieved aesthetic. I began with Mrs. Eck's story, and I close with a portrait of her, articulated by her son, Joe, and his partner, Wayne. Their e-mail dialogue with me is as unique and yet universally emblematic of family experience of being old and having cancer as Mrs. Eck's story is of that state and representative of the aesthetic sense of Mrs. Eck that they maintain throughout.

Joe Eck wrote of his mother, in reply to our mutual editor friend's query about whether Mrs. Eck might consent to speak to me of her experience:

Thank you for your interesting letter about Dr. Kagan's project. My response has to be a little complicated, but first I should say that I quickly see the importance of her work, and I hope it will round itself out in a wonderful way. My sisters and I think it might be possible for my mother to participate, but first I need to give you a small character sketch of her.

She is a first-generation American, my grandfather having left England when he was eighteen, returning (with us) not until he was eighty, to see three living siblings again for the first time in all the years between his departure and then. He was a rather fierce old man, who never showed any emotion in public, or demonstrated any affection, though he was passionately devoted to his two children, my mother and a sister, now deceased. His meeting with my great-aunt Nora was a case in point. No tears, no terms of endearment, no significant good-byes. But I know he was deeply moved.

I could hardly call my mother fierce, but she has certainly inherited my grandfather McIver's reticence, and his immense strength of character. He was a dam builder—an oddly significant profession—and he went out of retirement four times to assist on major projects throughout North America until he became too old to insure. My mother is very intelligent, a lifelong reader, and very committed to the world outside herself. She supports many charities, though always in the benefactors she is listed as "anonymous." She is very committed to all medical research, though when asked whether she would be willing to donate her organs after this illness had run its course, she said, "Aren't they all worn out?" When they said they essentially wanted the pancreas, she said, "Of course. You shouldn't have to ask." But only a few people call her by her first name.

I needed to draw this little portrait in order to explain why the word *cancer*, or even *death*, has never been used in her presence. She is not in denial; far from it. But all my life I have known that she could handle almost anything if a word was not put to it. Referring to *cancer* would somehow be unseemly, would call a kind of attention to herself she simply couldn't suffer.

The meals are one thing, because we are not actually sure what actual taste she has left. So food has become an idea, like so many things do with my mother. She has also had a new floor put down in the kitchen, has had all the woodwork freshly repainted, and she wants us to plant another Japanese maple in a quite precise corner of the front lawn, because the view beyond has always bothered her. She has her nails freshly painted, her hair done weekly, and she says about that: "I came into this world as a red-head and I am going out of it as a red-head." So jokes are possible; other things, perhaps not.

I am going down this weekend to help her make English fruit cakes, a family tradition. (When my grandfather died, he had fifteen of them, all from separate years, all faithfully bathed in good whiskey annually, and he never ate a one.) I will try to find an appropriate time to raise this question, or my sister Tracy will. I cannot exactly know what my mother will say. But if Dr. Kagan does succeed in interviewing her, she would need this information, since my mother can certainly turn frosty if anything is mentioned she considers "inappropriate." In every other way she is outgoing, hospitable, quite charming, and generous.

Joe presented my proposed visit to his mother and illuminated his report of her positive reply with further detail of her character:

I have just returned, as you know, from making Christmas fruit cakes with my mother. During the fiddle of that quite traditional process, I asked her if she would enjoy a visit from Sarah Kagan, and she said, "Actually, I would. I have been thinking about it. Just so long as she understands I am no scholar." That scholar part has occurred in our discussions before, and by it, I know my mother is simply expressing her instinctive modesty. She does not believe she has so much to offer on this subject. But she asked me, "What does she expect?" and I replied, "Candor, Mother." She then replied, "Oh. I think I can manage that." So if Dr. Kagan is still interested in her for a possible interview, I think the path is clear. I further think my mother would welcome Dr. Kagan's interest in her situation. Quite curiously, conversations between the two might be the only way in which she could express her actual feelings and seek information of a quite different sort from what her very cheerful doctors offer her. I should say, however, that in the year since this diagnosis was made, we have all seen a gradual sinking, so slow that it might be imperceptible except to the very attentive. This particular disease is supposed to be swift and relentless, and though we all accept the relentless part, the swift has been mercifully slow in coming. Still, we all seem to feel that the Holidays are probably the end of our reserves. So If Sarah wishes to speak to my mother, I would say it has to happen fairly soon. Our home town is an easy trip across the Bridge, in good traffic taking hardly fifteen minutes. Ours is just an old house in the suburbs, but maybe because I grew up there, I always feel that I am stepping back into the past, into something at once both deeply familiar and not quite like walking into any other front door. But my mother would want to have the carpet freshly vacuumed, and certainly she would want to have her hair and nails done. So some advance warning is important, but it appears we all are not expecting much at this point. Please forward this letter to Sarah if you think it might be useful to her. She should certainly write back to our e-mail address here if she has questions that might help her in her work. And if she wants to visit my mother, then we could help her plan the easiest time for both of them.

Our exchange continued as I arranged a visit at a time comfortable for Mrs. Eck. Joe wrote:

We can meet you ourselves, introduce you, make you a pot of tea and settle you both for your visit. We will then have some errands to do. But I am very sure my mother will enjoy this conversation, and will welcome you.

After this first visit everything will be easier. You will understand quickly that she is anxious with strangers, but at this point she is certainly not an invalid, and she enjoys company. She will give a thoughtful answer to almost any question. The two principal values of her life are her faith and her family. In this first conversation, it would be safest to start there. But my mother admires courage. So perhaps you should simply take a deep breath and plunge in. Forgive me if I seem officious here. I am sure you will know how to proceed.

I think an early afternoon visit would be best, just after lunch at around 1:00. Generally, she likes to nap around 3:30, but for all her life she has been committed to the idea that her own schedule and preferences should be arranged according to the needs of others. Still, talking with her at that time will be easiest, for her and we hope for you.

I had written again, just before the visit to confirm and ask what form of address Mrs. Eck preferred, and received a vivid reply:

We are all looking forward to meeting you. My mother seems to have entered a period of surprising strength. She had a wonderful holiday season, even walking to neighborhood parties and going out to a restaurant for her eighty-sixth birthday, which was yesterday. Her spirits are very strong, and her frailty comes really from a deteriorated hip which of course cannot be repaired, and not from her cancer. Of course, as you know, things can change quickly. But at present she is in no sense an invalid, and so you should not be anxious about over-staying your hour with her. Or perhaps, coming back to visit if that is useful to you, once you know the way. She will also not be at all disturbed by a notebook or tape recorder. She perfectly well understands the purpose of your visit, and has from the first. Given her age, I suppose one should start by calling her Mrs. Eck. She'll tell you if she prefers some other address.

Our dialogue lapsed and I guessed the reason—Mrs. Eck went from feeling well and energetic into a period of discomfort and necessary intervention. Wayne, Joe's partner, replied to my e-mail with images of Mrs. Eck as she transcended challenges common to pancreatic cancer:

We are sorry to have left your letter unanswered for so long. As you probably have surmised, for the last two weeks Joe's mother has had a difficult time. Travel [to see her]—with our own lecturing commitments—has left little time for writing. For the moment, however, things have stabilized, and so I am writing now.

Here is a quick summary of Mrs. Eck's situation. About a month ago she began to experience nausea and was unable to hold down food. A fourth stent was inserted, this time of metal rather than fiber, which we are told makes it the last one possible. That gave a brief respite, but two weeks after that the nausea returned, and her doctors discovered that her gall bladder was clogged. They cleaned it, and inserted another stent. She then began to complain of back pain, which was assumed to be kidney stones. Nausea and pain made it impossible to hold down food or water, so she was readmitted to the hospital. It turned out that there was a blockage in the kidney, so two days ago she signed herself back into surgery, and another stent has been inserted there. She is still in the hospital, but we assume she will be released today.

You might be amused by this small story. Day before yesterday, her urologist explained the kidney problem and scheduled surgery for next Monday. Then a slot opened, he offered it to her, she signed the papers immediately, and away she went. When Tracy, her youngest daughter, came for her morning visit, the room was empty. So Tracy began opening doors until she found Mrs. Eck in pre-op. The nurse there asked if Mrs. Eck was competent to sign herself in, and Tracy gave her a withering stare. "My mother pays all her bills herself and has just bought some real estate. I think therefore that she is QUITE competent."

We must assume that the pressure of the disease is now causing a collapse of the internal organs. It has been one year and three days since Mrs. Eck was first diagnosed with pancreatic cancer, and all that time has been a great gift. She has made excellent use of it, and as you saw, she has managed to maintain perfect philosophical balance and enjoy her days. Further, it has given others who love her—her husband particularly—time to adjust to the idea of her death, as far as one ever really can until it occurs. She has never complained and isn't complaining now. The inevitable humiliations of illness weigh heavily on her, for she has always been very conscious of her appearance and human dignity. But death has never seemed to frighten her, and doesn't, even now.

Mrs. Eck's gerontologist (whom you must know) has told her daughters that she has not yet reached the point where hospice care must take over. I think the implications of that statement, however, are that it will be soon. You may remember that Susan, her eldest daughter, is a highly skilled nurse with many connections in the medical community, and she will take leave from her work to assume most of the necessary care, which will be at home.

For the moment, there seems to be a brief respite, and that may be important to your own work. All of us, Mrs. Eck certainly included, would like to see it completed in a form that will be useful for your book. If this last intervention allows her to come home and be comfortable for a bit, I know that she would welcome a visit from you. She enjoyed her last talk with you immensely and has said so, many times.

I responded, wanting to remain distant enough to write of Mrs. Eck in a manner that would resonate with readers and simultaneously wishing in my clinical self to offer comfort from that distance:

Thank you so much for your very kind e-mail and for the explanation that I had imagined might be in the offing. I wanted to wait until I had Mrs. Eck's chapter—one that she and I thought would be titled "Hot Dogs and Champagne" in tribute to the lunch she enjoyed with her husband on so many Wednesdays—in better form. But I worried that she might experience some untoward events with the stent placement she mentioned when we met for tea. My prayers for a recovery that allows her to be at home with you all are constant. I agree that her gerontologist is foreshadowing what will come to be but that she may benefit from these interventions and enjoy her life without so many symptoms.

The detail with which you convey what Mrs. Eck is experiencing is vivid, and I almost feel as though I am there! I do especially appreciate the anecdote about signing herself in for surgery. May I say that this sort of thing is exactly why I want to write this book—it seems that we cannot see what is so deeply embedded and then act so illogically because of it. The assumption that older people are mentally incapable comes so quickly to so many! I wonder if I might use that episode in the book if I make it anonymous?

I am grateful for your thoughts of my work, the book, and the place of Mrs. Eck's story in it. Meeting her was a transcendent experience for me—though I hesitate to use such superlatives in daily description, they are fitting here. Mrs. Eck is at once every woman and yet so utterly, quintessentially, and uniquely herself. Her interview is representative of that wonderful character. I am almost finished putting it into chapter form. When we met, I had not formally asked her permission to use it finally as a chapter because I had wanted to outline the process and let her know that she would have a chance to review it before we decided anything. She had liked that plan, I think perhaps because time seemed to be less critical then than it is now. We did discuss details like a title, etc. as I mentioned earlier. I will e-mail Mrs. Eck's chapter to you as soon as it is drafted. In that way, you as a family will have it and you will also be able to show it to Mrs. Eck when she has interest. I would love to visit her again should that be possible. If it is not, I will confirm that in the event that Mrs. Eck cannot sign her permission, you as family can give permission on her behalf. I will e-mail a statement of permission with the chapter itself. I hope that will be at the end of this week or next. Does this plan sound agreeable to you?

In the meanwhile, know that my thoughts and prayers are with Mrs. Eck and with the family as you all enjoy time being together. More than anything, I am heartened to know she enjoyed our time together, as I did so as well. The force of her warmth and connection are, for me, considerable.

Wayne replied again, telling me of Mrs. Eck's ability to recover her footing and enjoy what she valued in daily life and of the family's response to her interview:

Don't thank us for our e-mails, your own being so generous and thoughtful. Because of your extensive experience, you will probably not be surprised that today's news is good. Mrs. Eck ate a good dinner, kept it down, finished a book, and is selecting a new one. Joe said, "Mother, shall I bring down some books?" and her reply was, "I have fifteen. That should last me my life, anyway." She is very comfortable, for the moment, but you well know one takes each day separately, and things change in a night.

We all think it very important for you to visit again, and that should be worked out if possible. Joe and I [will visit] on the twenty-first, and if your schedule permitted, and Mrs. Eck is well enough to have a guest, that might be possible. But though we would like very much to see you again, we are not really necessary, and if your schedule demanded an earlier date, it could possibly be arranged. Joe will speak with her tonight (He does every night, since the diagnosis) and ask what she would like. Obviously, too, a call the morning of your visit would be necessary, given the volatile nature of this stage of the disease. . . .

We certainly agree with you that Mrs. Eck is a remarkable woman, but actually, nothing about the way she has handled this illness is out of character in the least. I should tell you also that she possesses the English reserve of her father, a fierce old gentleman, and if she hadn't liked you—which she richly did—you would have found her quite frosty. "Formally polite" might be a better way to put it.

I hope your book is going well, midst all your other commitments. And please let us help in any way we can. By "we," I mean not only Joe and me, but Mrs. Eck's three daughters, all remarkable in their separate ways. And Mr. Eck has been magnificent, we think, both in the care he has given and the resignation he has achieved, which none of us expected.

Wayne mentions Mrs. Eck's formality as well as the understanding of all involved that her interview would not be recast in hindsight. How true that prediction was, as Mrs. Eck reviewed the transcript with me and seemed thoroughly engaged. She had only one request, a small change in manner of speech, a mannerism on which we both relied and both disliked seeing in print. I assured Mrs. Eck that I would edit the transcript so that it was removed from both our voices. It is our private exchange and one that bound her to me rather personally.

I visited Mrs. Eck that second time and received an e-mail from Joe afterward:

It was a great pleasure seeing you last Tuesday, and my mother hugely enjoyed her visit with you. She has read the rough draft of your chapter, and she is pleased by it except for one small detail. [Joe wrote then with humor and kindness of the manner of speech that Mrs. Eck and I both disliked in ourselves on reading the transcript—a matter I keep private between Mrs. Eck and myself—and notes that she vows to change it for the rest of her life.] Under the present circumstances, I think she can keep to that. Is it possible to make that one small change? I would like to tell her so, as she seems to be fretful about it.

We returned to New York on Wednesday, and on Thursday morning we got the news that she had been readmitted to Smith Hospital with massive internal bleeding. Investigations made clear that there are many ulcers, mostly in the esophagus, an inevitable consequence, we assume, of so many interventions and drugs. She is still in intensive care, and the bleeding has mostly stopped. We assume—though with your expertise you may know better—that we are very near the end. With my mother, however, one could not possibly say. She has, after all, lived fourteen months after this diagnosis, and she may yet surprise us. She is as you last saw her, gallant, cheerful, humorous, and patient. She possesses a calmness in the face of all this that fills us with awe. If she has any discomfort at all, it is in the inevitable bodily humiliations of the disease, for she has always been fastidious and immaculate in her person. But even that she seems able to bear with an astonishing degree of stoicism.

Wayne and I are returning tomorrow, though we are only able to remain for one day, unless we learn that we must stay longer. If in this last phase there is anything we could do to further your work, please do not hesitate to ask. My mother has signed the release forms and emphatically prefers not to remain anonymous. "Why would I want that?" she said, with genuine puzzlement.

I replied and received a last response from Wayne before our correspondence closed and they focused their energies on Mrs. Eck as she entered hospice care:

It is my turn to answer, now. As always, we are grateful for so long and thoughtful a letter from you. It has some specific questions for which you need answers, and I will give them in a bit. But we wanted you to know the current state of Joe's mother's health, and her progress.

Her time in the emergency ward was tense, but quiet. Her principal doctor felt it very important to get her home, and that was of course her wish also. And ours, since it is impossible to surround her with pretty things and smells in a hospital, but easy in her own home. A bed has been moved into the sun room, just off the parlor, in fact in the very spot where her own mother died, forty-eight years ago. This is of course a conjunction that is meaningful to her, in a deep way. All her children . . . have been around her, and we go down tomorrow, for two days. Someone is with her around the clock, and we will take our turns at that, giving the others a break.

I think Mrs. Eck feels a tiny bit of renaissance—or maybe even triumph—in surviving to get home once more. She said, indeed, when she was driven up the drive, "I just thought I would never see my house again." We are all hoping that some crisis will not put her back into emergency care again, though that is certainly a possibility. She has had two bouts with congestive heart failure, and her blood sugar level is very unstable. Eating, we all understand, is essential, but that is difficult for her. She has no pain, which is of course a blessing, though it means that hospice cannot intervene. So we wait, from day to day, meal to meal.

I am about to speculate, Sarah, in a subject you know so very well. Forgive me if I am stupid. But I think in these tough and courageous women there is a very strong will to live. The panoply of strategies they employ to cope with their illness, which you are presently chronicling, helps in that. They seem to want to hold on—or at least I can say that Mrs. Eck does—just because they are courageous, and committed to "doing a good job." The resignation necessary to turn loose, to give in, to submit, is just not in them. It seems like a lack of character. And it reflects a form of denial more subtle than we had realized. It isn't denial of the fact of death, which is assured; it is a denial of NOW. One more day becomes a goal. I am sure that the weariness of pain, or of radical interventions to sustain life, might be a kind of permission to quit. But that has not happened yet.

Wayne's words closed my interlude with Mrs. Eck and opened for me a new way of considering a tension unique to being old when viewed from a position of youth. The gradual diminution of that sense of immortality we have and need when we are young does not result in a frank welcoming of death and comfort with dying. Wayne's observations of Mrs. Eck's death highlighted something I had observed in both my personal and professional lives. Given the chance in later life, people will often deny death now without denying their own proximate mortality to complete living. Once living is done or when living is unbalanced by unacceptable suffering, death is more often accepted as a "now." I admire that capacity to gauge living and death for oneself that accrues in late life.

Postscript
Completed

At the very end of August 2006, as I pounded away—literally, with finger strikes that clattered on my computer keyboard—at what I hoped would be final edits to the manuscript for this book, I received an e-mail titled succinctly "Completed." I was taken aback by the superficial coincidence. As I completed effortful writing incorporating what I had learned from her, Mrs. Eck had more momentously completed her life a few hours earlier. Joe's partner, Wayne, had written the message, voicing memory and mourning, with an eloquence I could only hope to reach:

That's a bit of a dramatic heading, I suppose, but we did want you to know that Joe's mother died early this morning, at Stein Hospital. We had seen her the week before and brought her a Hermes scarf, for till the very end her hair was done and her nails fresh and painted, and because of extreme weight loss, she had resumed a remarkable girlish prettiness. All her other children were with her last night, and Susan, who is an experienced nurse, was in charge. Even at the end, she [Mrs. Eck] simply didn't seem to want to give up.

We have thought of writing you, many times during these last months. The illness has gone on an extraordinary length of time for pancreatic cancer—as you can calculate—almost 19 months. During all that time there has been no pain until this week, though the decline has been steady. Mrs. Eck was in and out of the hospital, as one function or another began to fail. Many stents have been inserted, into the gall bladder, into one kidney, even in small sections down her throat. This last crisis was an inability to urinate, and that was corrected, briefly, by a massive transfusion of blood and by renewing some of the stents.

For some weeks she has been unable to eat, and has been fed intravenously. Though she has had a day nurse, one or another of her children has spent the night near her. Restless nights, because her mouth has dried, and she has craved ice chips, essentially the only thing she could ingest. So there was a call every hour through the night. Her daughter Tracy, who is witty, said, "Mom, my name used to be Tracy. Now it's Ice Chips."

Of course, no one resented this care. Some of us—well . . . I, at least . . . did have a question of why she was choosing to go through so many interventions, all very stressful for a lady of eighty-six years. Her doctors have loved her, for her courage and her wit, and their encouragement and even their pure medical interest in such a case have kept her going. (She once ruefully referred to herself as their white rat.) When one's doctors tell one that one is brave, and that they will stick by you as long as you want to fight, that is certainly an encouragement.

But I think there were other things involved. Religious faith for one, though I myself do not possess it, controls one's actions, our "ought to," and if it is strong, to the very last. I think that to have opted for some easy solution would simply have seemed to Mrs. Eck a mortal sin, tantamount to suicide. When one adds to that her sense of duty, which did after all raise five children and keep a very complex house going, it doesn't seem strange that she would see the job to its end, just simply as something that had to be done.

Beyond all that—which is certainly a lot—I think she was actually amused by it all. Her mind and her sense of wit and irony remained keen almost to the very end, and I think she would have said at any dire point, "Well, here's a fine mess!"

I am putting a good face on this loss, but I should certainly acknowledge the sadness that is left by it. We leave tomorrow, and the funeral, so far as we know, will be on Thursday. It will all be hard. And left behind is her husband, also eighty-six, who is going, in his turn, to be some hard work. We are all taking deep breaths.

There are so many layers to a final parting, Sarah, and the deepest is that one mourns for oneself, for one's own mortality, and wonders how it will be, and, if the job is in one's own hands, how one will do it, and how well. That's only just to say that these events face us with the truth. We take that truth in fits and starts, until—lucky or unlucky—we have to take the whole thing.

I replied simply:

Thank you for your e-mail. In complete and startling coincidence, your message finds me at my computer today, polishing the final bits of the now completed manuscript. I struggled for months to finish it, for reasons you and Joe will likely see especially manifest in the introduction. In truth, it was only looking like a book last week. It is really only in that form because of Mrs. Eck and her consolidating influence on me and my writing. In fact, she and the book were with me day and night since I last spoke with her and sorted through her incredible interview and the effects it had on my thinking. It is then because of Mrs. Eck that the book is complete and, I hope, of use to some audience. She gave me most generous gift in the short time that I knew her. I hope that her gift to me will help others who read our now conjoined stories.

Mrs. Eck is truly and profoundly, as your description of her final months and days attests, an astounding and transcendent woman. She is most certainly present, and then written of in the present tense, as she lives in my memory and my writing as I'm sure she lives in the memories of all who love her and know her. I am deeply grateful to Joe, you, and her extended family for sharing her with me, as I am to Mrs. Eck for giving of herself. Words are clearly not enough at a time such as this. Please know though that my thoughts and prayers are with you all. I wish you all peace in the coming months, serenity in Mrs. Eck's memory, and joy in wonderful memories of her.

As with other older people whom I have known and those for whom I have been privileged to provide care, Mrs. Eck—as one of the most endearing and indelible personalities I have encountered—taught me more than I could possibly have given to her. The knowledge she gave me is a gift, a gift that I in turn attempt to bequeath in writing, in care for those who are old and have cancer and for those who care about and for them.

Notes

Introduction

1. My deep appreciation to Rebecca Trotta for extensive conversation on this topic, as she analyzed for her doctoral work the trajectory of dying displayed in the literature.

2. *Embodiment* is a philosophically oriented term I use to describe the situation of inhabiting one's body as a whole, integrated person without division between mind and body. Embodiment is often best captured in considering a skill—such as driving a car or playing a game like soccer—that requires the mind and body to be entirely and comprehensively integrated.

3. See http://www.eifoundation.org/national/nccra/splash/.

4. See http://www.eifoundation.org/press/release.asp?press_release_id=47.

Chapter 1

1. All institutional names used in this chapter have been changed.

2. The clinicians' names used in this chapter have been changed.

Chapter 2

1. See Chapter 5 for further discussion of this equation, which I label "quality of daily living," as opposed to the ordinary global measurement "quality of life," which is uniformly employed in health care research and practice.

2. This name is a pseudonym.

3. This study was funded by the Fellowship in Clinical Qualitative Gero-Oncology Nursing Research, Oncology Nursing Foundation/Hoechst-Marion Roussel, September 1996–March 1999.

Chapter 3

1. The crawl appeared on 1 February 2005. A discussion of the scientific paper on quercetin appears in the article entitled Apples May Ward Off Alzheimer's Disease: Antioxidant in Apples Helps Protect Brain Cells in Lab Test by Miranda Hitti; http://my.webmd.com/content/article/97/104093.htm, accessed on 2 February 2005.

2. On the origin of the apple-a-day saying, see http://www.famousquotes.me.uk/nursery_rhymes/an_apple_a_day.htm and http://www.school-for-champions.com/biographies/franklin.htm.

3. The Hayflick limit is, most simply, the idea that cells cultured in a Petri dish will grow and divide a certain number of times and then die. The Hayflick limit is fundamentally important to scientific understandings of the aging process in that it shows that cells themselves age. It is also connected to the biology of cancer as a reverse condition.

4. The text of *Rip Van Winkle* is available online at http://www.bartleby.com/195/4.html.

5. Titian, *The Three Ages of Man*, 1513–14, oil on canvas, 90 × 151 cm, National Gallery of Scotland, Edinburgh.

Chapter 4

This chapter is based on a talk given at the University of Pennsylvania Institute on Aging twenty-fifth anniversary retreat, May 2004, in Philadelphia, Pennsylvania. See also Chapter 3.

1. My thanks to Anna Song Beeber, with whom I have engaged in extended conversation on dependence, independence, and interdependence.

Chapter 5

The work represented in this chapter was funded in part by the Trustees' Council of Penn Women Summer Research Fellowship, Fellowship in Clinical Qualitative Gero-Oncology Nursing Research; Oncology Nursing Foundation/Hoechst-Marion Roussel, September; Pre-Doctoral Fellow, National Research Service Award, Institutional Grant #T32-AG00130, "Training in Gerontological Nursing Research"; Sigma Theta Tau Alpha Eta Chapter Research Funds; Century Club Funds, The University of California, San Francisco; and Graduate Division Funds, The University of California, San Francisco. This chapter is developed from a talk titled "Language Lessons Learned from Older Adults with Cancer: Merging Grounded Theory and Practice" at 6:e Nationella Konferensen I Cancervård (Annual Meeting of the Swedish Cancer Nurses Society) in Stockholm, Sweden in April 2004. The author is indebted to Carol Tishelman, Lena Sharp, and Britt-Marie Bernhardson for their introduction to the Swedish Cancer Nurses Society and for their rewarding colleagueship. The author is grateful for the support of Meg Wallhagen, Juliet Corbin, and DeLois Weekes of original works that form the foundation of this chapter.

1. Please see Chapter 4.

2. War and battle in cancer are most vividly and popularly portrayed, to the end of vast social benefit, by the phenomenon of Lance Armstrong's triumph over testicular cancer and the manner in which his survival and subsequent Tour de France victories are parlayed into philanthropic bounty in the Lance Armstrong Foundation. See the "About Us" section of the foundation Web site, http://www.livestrong.org/site/c.khLXK1PxHmF/b.2660611/k.BCED/Home.

htm: "We believe that unity is strength, knowledge is power and attitude is everything."

Chapter 6

An original version of this chapter was supported by a grant from the Frank Morgan Jones Fund at the University of Pennsylvania and presented at the International Council of Nurses Centennial Meeting, London, June 1999. The original paper, as the foundation, and hence this chapter are coauthored by Ara A. Chalian. We gratefully acknowledge the significant support, insightful intellectual critique, and thoughtful guidance of E. Ann Matter, Julie S. Fairman, and Mary Beth Happ in preparing the original paper.

1. See http://www.webwhispers.org/ and http://www.spohnc.org/.

References

Babbitt, N. 1985. *Tuck everlasting.* New York: Farrar, Straus, and Giroux.

Bridger, A. G., C. J. O'Brien, and K. K. Lee. 1994. Advanced patient age should not preclude the use of free-flap reconstruction for head and neck cancer. *American Journal of Surgery* 168:425–27.

Bruns, B. 2004. Joe Napolitano: Full of zest at 105. *Palisadian-Post* [Pacific Palisades, Calif.]. http://www.palisadespost.com/content/index.cfm?Story_ID=580 (accessed 4 August 2005).

Cole, Thomas R. 1992. *The journey of life: A cultural history of aging in America.* Cambridge, UK: Cambridge University Press.

Cutler, D. M., and E. Meara. 1997. *The medical costs of the young and old: A forty year perspective.* Cambridge, Mass.: National Bureau of Economic Research. http://papers.nber.org/papers/W6114 (accessed 11 January 2005).

Donaldson, M. S. 2004. Taking stock of health-related quality of life measurement in oncology practice in the United States. *Journal of the National Cancer Institute Monographs* 33:155–67.

Ferri, C. P., M. Prince, C. Brayne, H. Brodaty, L. Fratiglioni, M. Ganguli, K. Hall, K. Hasegawa, H. Hendrie, and Y. Huang. 2005. Global prevalence of dementia: A Delphi consensus study. *Lancet* 366 (9503):2112–17.

Haiken, E. 1994. Plastic surgery and American beauty at 1921. *Bulletin of the History of Medicine* 68:429–53.

———. 2000. The making of the modern face: Cosmetic surgery. *Social Research* 67 (1):81–97.

Hall, S. S. 2003. *Merchants of immortality.* New York: Houghton Mifflin.

Hazzard, W. R. 1997. Ways to make "usual" and "successful" aging synonymous: Preventive gerontology. *Western Journal of Medicine* 167 (4):206–15.

Himes, C. L. 2003. *Age 100 and counting.* Washington, D.C.: Population Reference Bureau. http://www.prb.org/Template.cfm?Section=PRB&template=/ContentManagement/ContentDisplay.cfm&ContentID=8420 (accessed 11 January 2005).

Jemal, A., T. Murray, E. Ward, A. Samuels, R. C. Tiwari, A. Ghafoor, E. J. Feuer, and M. J. Thun. 2005. Cancer Statistics, 2005. *CA: A Cancer Journal for Clinicians* 55 (1):10–30.

Kagan, S. H. 1994. Integrating cancer into a life mostly lived (elderly). Unpublished diss.

———. 1997. *Older adults coping with cancer: Integrating cancer into a life mostly lived; Aging in America.* New York: Garland.

———. 2004. Gero-oncology nursing research. *Oncology Nursing Forum* 31 (2):293–99.

Kearney, N., M. Miller, J. Paul, and K. Smith. 2000. Oncology healthcare professionals' attitudes toward elderly people. *Annals of Oncology* 11 (5):599–601.

Lee, R., and J. Skinner. 1999. Will aging baby boomers bust the federal budget? *Journal of Economic Perspectives* 13 (1):117–40.

Leichter, H. M. 2003. "Evil habits" and "personal choices": Assigning responsibility for health in the 20th century. *Milbank Quarterly* 81 (4):603–26.

Levy, B. 1996. Improving memory in old age through implicit self-stereotyping. *Journal of Personality & Social Psychology* 71 (6):1092–1107.

Levy, B., O. Ashman, and I. Dror. 1999. To be or not to be: The effects of aging stereotypes on the will to live. *Omega Journal of Death & Dying* 40 (3):409–20.

Levy, B., and E. Langer. 1994. Aging free from negative stereotypes: Successful memory in China and among the American deaf. *Journal of Personality & Social Psychology* 66 (6):989–97.

Levy, B. R. 1999. The inner self of the Japanese elderly: A defense against negative stereotypes of aging. *International Journal of Aging & Human Development* 48 (2):131–44.

———. 2001. Eradication of ageism requires addressing the enemy within. *Gerontologist* 41 (5):578–79.

———. 2003. Mind matters: Cognitive and physical effects of aging self-stereotypes. *Journals of Gerontology Series B Psychological Sciences & Social Sciences* 58 (4):203–11.

Lieber, J. 2002. *Tuck everlasting.* Ed. J. Russell. (Film.) Los Angeles: Beacon Pictures (formerly Beacon Communications).

Mead, G. H. 1967. *Mind, self, and society: From the standpoint of a social behaviorist (works of George Herbert Mead).* Ed. C. W. Morris. Chicago: University of Chicago Press.

Miller, M. 1999. Ageism within cancer care: A priority for nursing. *European Journal of Oncology Nursing* 3 (1):25–30.

Munnell, A. H. 2004. Population aging: It's not just the baby boom. *In Brief: Center for Retirement Research at Boston College,* issue in brief 16. Available online at http://crr.bc.edu/images/stories/Briefs/ib_16.pdf?phpMyAdmin=43ac48 3c4de9t51d9eb4.

Napolitano, J. 2005. *About Joe Napolitano, 105. Palisadian-Post* [Pacific-Palisades, Calif.]. http://www.palisadespost.com/content/index.cfm?Story_ID=1087 (accessed 4 August 2005).

Olson, M. L., and D. P. Shedd. 1978. Disability and rehabilitation in head and neck cancer patients after treatment. *Head and Neck Surgery* 1:52–58.

Patterson, J. T. 1987. *The dread disease: Cancer and modern American culture.* Cambridge, Mass.: Harvard University Press.

Petersen, B. 2005. Buicks in China. *CBS Sunday Morning.* New York: CBS Television.

Repetto, L., and L. Balducci. 2002. A case for geriatric oncology. *Lancet Oncology* 3 (5):289–97.

Rowe, J. W., and R. L. Kahn. 1987. Human aging: Usual and successful. *Science* 237 (4811):143–49.

Schuman, H. and Rodgers, W. L. 2004. Cohorts, chronology, and collective memories. *Public Opinion Quarterly* 68 (2):217–55.

Scommegna, P. 2004. *U.S. growing bigger, older, and more diverse.* Washington, D.C.: Population Reference Bureau. http://www.prb.org/Template.cfm?Section=PR B&template=/ContentManagement/ContentDisplay.cfm&ContentID=10201 (accessed 11 January 2005).

Sporn, M. B. 1996. The war on cancer. *Lancet* 347 (9012):1377–81.

Yancik, R., and L. A. Ries. 2000. Aging and cancer in America: Demographic and epidemiologic perspectives. *Hematology: Oncology Clinics of North America* 14 (1):17–23.

Index

aesthetics of being old and having cancer, 76–86; and age and gender considerations in clinical treatment, 81–82, 84–86; and breast cancer, 7, 76–77, 79–83; and colorectal cancer, 79; and competing social images, 81; head and neck cancers, 6–7, 8, 78–86; how cancer alters embodiment, 77–78; and lung cancer, 79; moral interpretations, 80; and personal experience of living in an aging body, 77; and prostate cancer, 79; and reconstructive surgery decisions, 82–86; religious and cultural views of morality and cancer, 76, 80; and shifts in treatment paradigms, 76–77. *See also* sociocultural meanings of being old and having cancer

age, chronological: and age discrimination, 58–60, 63, 67; and socially mediated constructions of old age, 14–15, 31, 33, 53, 58–60, 66–67; and treatment decisions, 63

age and cancer risk, 1–2

age considerations in clinical treatment of cancer, 81–82, 84–86

age discrimination (ageism), 58–60, 63, 66–67; and clinicians, 66–67; in family contexts (speaking for one's parent), 59; "granny" bashing, 58, 59; and language of chronological age, 59–60, 67; reverse parentalism, 58–59; self-stereotyping, 58–59; senility stereotypes, 59; and treatment decisions, 59–60, 63

Alzheimer's disease, 31, 39–40, 57

"antiaging" science, 39–40

Armstrong, Lance, 61, 100n.2

baby boom generation, 45, 60–61

battles against cancer, 18, 25–27, 71, 100n.2. *See also* war on cancer

biomedical notions of disease and old age, 30–31. *See also* science

blessings, 22–24

breast cancer, 5, 7; and aesthetics, 7, 76–77, 79–83; and glamorization of survivorship, 61; media coverage and public awareness, 7, 8, 77, 80–81; and reconstructive surgery decisions, 82–83; treatment paradigms and distortion of self-image, 76–77

capacity/incapacity and distress in illness, 33

Chalian, Ara, 6

clinical trials, 47

clinicians (physicians): and age discrimination, 66–67; and prognostication, 2–3; "symptom stories," 73–74; views of older adults' participation in their health care, 66; and voice and power in health care, 66–67

colorectal cancer, 5, 7, 79

Couric, Katie, 7

Cristofalo, Vincent, 40

demographics of health care and aging population, 52–53

digestive tract cancers, 5, 7; colorectal cancer, 5, 7, 79; media coverage and public awareness, 7–8. *See also* pancreatic cancer

The Dread Disease: Cancer and Modern American Culture (Patterson), 29

Eck, Joe, 1–2, 8, 87–97

Eck, Mrs., 1–3, 7–8, 9–24, 25–26, 36, 71,

Eck, Mrs. (*continued*)
87–97; author's first meeting with, 1–3, 9–24, 87–90; on being asked about her final plans/belongings, 13, 19; on being offered treatment choices, 11; blocked bile duct and stent procedures, 10–14, 90, 95; on confidence in/discomfort with doctors' approaches, 11–12, 15; contemplation of her blessings, 22–24; death, 95–97; declining health, 90–91, 93–94; on experiences of others' kindness, 21–22; on "fighting a battle" against cancer, 18, 71; happiness/positive outlook, 18, 21–23, 96; hip replacement issue, 9–10, 12, 19; itching and jaundice, 10, 14; living with her diagnosis, 13, 18–19, 94; maintaining a personal style, 15, 23–24, 88, 92; marriage, 15–16, 17–18, 23; on overhearing physicians discuss her prognosis, 2–3, 10, 19, 26; pain and medications, 13; preoperative testing and diagnostic surgery, 11–12; on radiation and chemotherapy, 12, 19–20; reminiscence about her sister, 16–17, 20–21; sense of family, 13, 22–23; son's character sketch of, 87–88; use of language/words *cancer* and *death*, 88
embodiment, 33–34, 77–78, 99n.2
Entertainment Industry Foundation, 7

failure: and language of cancer treatment, 47–48, 63–64; successful aging and moral implications of, 32–33
families and cancer, 2; and care needs, 53; reverse parentalism and speaking for one's parent, 59
"fountain of youth" and immortality, 40–44

gastrointestinal cancers. *See* digestive tract cancers; pancreatic cancer
gender considerations in clinical treatment of cancer, 81–82, 84–86
generalist health care, 46
genomic science, 50
gerontology: bench scientists and cellular senescence, 40, 41; and generalist health care, 46; language of successful aging/usual aging, 32, 36
glamorization of cancer survivorship, 601

Grant, Ulysses S., 29
gynecological cancers, 5

Hall, Stephen, 40–41, 43–44
Hayflick limit, 41, 43–44, 100n.3
Hazzard, W. R., 32
head and neck cancers, 5–8; as aesthetically unlike other cancers, 78–81; and aesthetics, 6–7, 8, 78–86; age and gender considerations in clinical treatment, 81–82, 84–86; and competing social images, 81; and morality, 80; reconstructive surgery decisions, 82–86; relative obscurity of, 80–81
Hospital of the University of Pennsylvania, 6

immortality, 40–44
"integrating cancer into a life mostly lived," 65, 69, 70–72; as alternative to metaphor of war on cancer, 71, 100n.2; as basic psychological process, 70–71; and framing of clinical care, 72; and sense of proximate mortality, 69, 70–71, 94; situating cancer in context of life rather than death, 71–72
Irving, Washington, 43

Kahn, R. L., 32

language and the experience of living with cancer, 65–75; battle language, 18, 25–27, 71, 100n.2; clinicians and age discrimination, 66–67; concept of "integrating cancer into a life mostly lived," 65, 69, 70–72; concept of "quality of daily living," 34–36, 48, 65, 69–70, 74–75; concept of "symptom stories," 65, 69, 72–74; and personal narratives, 62–63, 64; present-tense evaluations of daily life, 34–36, 70; success/failure and language of cancer treatment, 47–48, 63–64; voice and power in health care, 66–67
laryngectomy, 84
life expectancy, 30
living with cancer. *See* "integrating cancer into a life mostly lived"; language and the experience of living with cancer; "quality of daily living"; surviving cancer
longevity, individual reactions to the desire for, 41–43

lung cancer, 5, 29, 79

"mature generation," 45–46
media coverage and public awareness of cancer, 7, 8, 39–40, 80–81
melanoma and other skin cancers, 2–5
Merchants of Immortality (Hall), 40–41, 43–44
"middle age," 56–57
mind-body Cartesian dualism, 56–57
morality and cancer, 28–30; and aesthetic interpretations of head and neck cancers, 80; implications of failure, 32–33; personal behavior and responsibility, 29–30, 56; and Protestant tradition, 28, 29, 56, 76, 80; and successful aging, 28, 29, 32–33, 56; and tobacco consumption, 27, 28–29, 56, 62
mortality. *See* proximate mortality

Napolitano, Joe, 34–35, 36
narratives of being old and having cancer, 62–63, 64. *See also* Eck, Mrs.
National Colorectal Cancer Research Alliance, 7
Nixon, Richard, 38, 47
nursing: author's practice, 4, 5–7; and care needs/intimacy of care, 53–54; head and neck cancers, 6–7

Older Adults Coping with Cancer: Integrating Cancer into a Life Mostly Lived (Kagan), 2
"old-old" population, 45–46, 52–53

pancreatic cancer, 5, 7–8; detection and diagnoses, 7; media coverage and public awareness, 7–8; Mrs. Eck's preoperative testing and diagnostic surgery, 11–12; Mrs. Eck's stent procedures, 10–14, 90, 95
paradoxes of cancer and aging, 38–48; cancer as cognitive puzzle, 38; cellular senescence, 40, 41; discourse linking youth and consumption/consumer goods, 44–45; dissonance between our imaginings and the realities, 44; language of survival/failure pervading cancer care, 47–48, 63–64; link between old age and cancer, 38; news media and "antiaging" science, 39–40; and the quality of daily living, 48; quests

for "fountain of youth" (immortality), 40–44; schism between diagnosis and death, 47–48; societal focus on baby boomers' aging, 45, 60–61; struggle between inevitability of aging and the science that hopes to mitigate it, 39–40, 47–48; study and practice in aging and the notion of aging as non-normative, 46
parentalism, reverse, 58–59
Patterson, J. T., 29
possession of cancer/disease, 63
prognoses, 2–3
prostate cancer, 5, 79
Protestant tradition, 28, 29, 56, 76, 80
proximate mortality, 55, 62; and concept of "integrating cancer into a life mostly lived," 69, 70–71, 94; and the quality of daily living, 48; and social constructions of having cancer, 55, 62

"quality of daily living," 34–36, 48, 65, 69–70, 74–75; and interplay between past, present, and future in age-related illness, 34–36; present-tense evaluations, 34–36, 70; and proximate mortality, 48; and "quality of life" assessments by questions and retrospective time frame, 69–70; and reconstructive surgery decisions, 82–83; use in clinical care, 74
quercetin (antioxidant), 39–40

reconstructive surgery, 82–86; and age and gender considerations, 85–86; and breast cancer, 82–83; and disfigurement from wartime casualties, 83–84; head and neck cancers, 82–86
Rip Van Winkle story, 43
Rowe, J. W., 32

science: and "antiaging," 39–40; appraisals of progress in, 51; balance between creativity and continuity in, 51; biomedical notions of disease and old age, 30–31; and continua of human body systems (aging as biological progression), 57; as human enterprise/social phenomenon, 50–52; human interactions and paradigms in, 51–52; political nature and social context, 50; received views of, 51; and socially constructed understand-

science (*continued*)
    ings of being old and having cancer, 49, 57–58, 60–62; value in, 50
self-stereotyping, 58–59
senility stereotypes, 59
sinus cancer, 35–36
sociocultural meanings of being old and having cancer, 25–37, 49, 52–64; aging and evolving relationships, 54–55; aging as biological progression/disease as natural aspect of aging, 57; and behaviors contradicting socially mediated constructions, 31–32; biomedicine, 30–31; cancer and an individual's personal history, 25–26, 27–28; capacity/incapacity and distress in illness, 33; and chronological age, 31, 33, 53, 58–60, 66–67; competing metaphors of activity and attractiveness, 60–61; dichotomies of aging, 56–57; disgust and fear, 29; dying of "old age," 32–33; and embodiment, 33–34, 77–78, 99n.2; glamorization of cancer survivorship, 61; historical themes, 55–56; and individual narratives, 62–63, 64; inherently negative constructions, 62; interplay between past, present, and future in age-related illness, 34–36; morality and disease, 27, 28–30, 32–33, 56, 76, 80; notions of independence and dependence, 53; notions of lost function and ensuing need for care, 53–54; outdated constructions, 55; and physical and mental fitness, 28, 31; pity, 27; and Protestant tradition, 28, 29, 56, 76, 80; stereotypes of debility, despair, and death, 25, 26–27; and success and failure, 32–33, 47–48, 63–64; "successful aging," 28, 29, 32–33, 36, 56; temporal expectations of personal proximate mortality, 55, 62; tensions between scientific and social constructions, 49, 57–58, 60. *See also* aesthetics of being old and having cancer
successful aging: gerontological language of, 32, 36; and implications of failure, 32–33; and morality, 28, 29, 32–33, 56; and physical and mental fitness, 28; Protestant Christian images of, 28, 29

suffering, individual notions of, 61–62
Support for People with Oral and Head and Neck Cancer (SPOHNC), 81
surviving cancer: glamorization of, 61; language of survival and failure pervading cancer care, 47–48, 63–64; public phenomenon of living with cancer, 5
"symptom management," 69, 72, 73
"symptom stories," 65, 69, 72–74; and clinicians, 73–74; as iterative cycle of stories, 72–74; and resolution (incomplete/complete), 72, 73–74; and "symptom management," 69, 72, 73

temporal expectations of mortality, 55, 62. *See also* proximate mortality
testicular cancer, 61, 100n.2
Titian, *The Three Ages of Man*, 46–47
tobacco use: and lung cancer, 29, 79; and morality and immorality, 27, 28–29, 56, 62, 80
Tuck Everlasting (Babbitt), 43

University of Pennsylvania Institute on Aging, 40
usual aging, 32, 36

war on cancer: and aesthetics of being old and having cancer, 84; and Armstrong, 100n.2; battles on many fronts, 26–27; and concept of "integrating cancer into a life mostly lived," 71; language of battle, 18, 25–27, 71, 100n.2; Mrs. Eck's "battle," 18, 71; and Nixon, 38, 47; and struggle between inevitability of aging and the science that hopes to mitigate it, 38, 47–48; wartime casualties and disfigurement/reconstructive surgery, 83–84
WebWhispers Nu-Voice Club, 81

youth: and consumption/consumer goods, 44–45; quests for "fountain of youth," 40–44; and young-old dichotomy of aging, 56–57

Acknowledgments

This book is a funny thing: it is an inanimate object with which I have dwelled far too long and simultaneously a virtual place of discourse in which strands of thought come together through conversation with people from across my personal and professional lives. My parents, Nancy and Ralph, formed a backdrop that supported my writing. My brother, Joshua, and his wife, Abigail, were always encouraging and enthusiastic. I am grateful for the conversations with my friends and colleagues: Julie Fairman, whose own adventures in writing offered me much-needed camaraderie; Cheryl Boberick, Mary Denno, and Nancy Rodenhausen, for clinical conversations that flipped analysis back to reality; Ann Matter, Neville Strumpf, and Karen Wilkerson for sagacious counsel; Janice Foust and Meg Bourbonniere, who offered funny pep talks when I complained too much; Mary Beth Happ, for always keen insights; Ara Chalian, who provided intellectual engagement that helped me shape central aspects of the book; and my then doctoral students with whom I often had long conversations relevant to the chapter of the moment, Eunice Suh, Margaret Crighton, and Anna Beeber. My editor, Jo Joslyn at the University of Pennsylvania Press, introduced me to Mrs. Eck through her son, Joe, and his partner, Wayne. Their collective generosity altered the trajectory of this book. I am indebted to Renee Fox for her generous counsel and for seeing the book and my work in a light I could not. Alicia Puppione and Carrie Stricker helped me integrate Renee's reaction to the book, spending precious time in the summer of 2007 ripping apart what needed revision. I finally pulled it together with their help. My former student Sarah Strauss stepped in with great energy and a sharp eye to get the manuscript into its finished form. And, with a last minute request, Lorna McGonigal and Christine Ray rescued me by helping to revise the title.